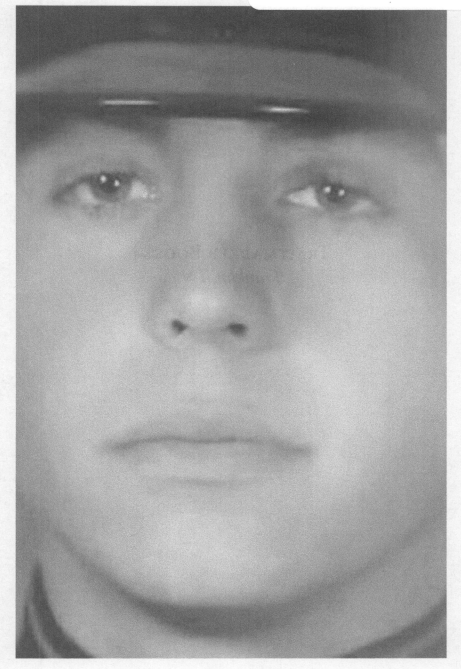

TRAITMARKER BOOKS |
Franklin, TN

Live to Tell

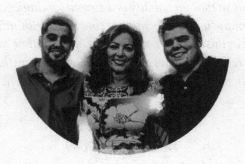

*The Fatal Consequences of
Pharmaceutical Suicide
and the Way Forward*

MAMA LUTZ

Traitmarker Books
2984 Del Rio Pike
Franklin, TN 37069
traitmarkerbooks.com
traitmarker@gmail.com

Interior Text Font: Minion Pro
Interior Title Fonts: Minion Pro
Editor: Sharilyn Grayson
Cover Design: Robbie Grayson III

ISBN 978-1-0879-8240-3
Printed in the United States of America

pharmaceutical-induced suicide \ n

1: death by suicide directly caused by neurotoxic chemicals within prescription drugs that derail personal choice and healthy thought | 2: death caused by prescription drugs hijacking a person's will and thought process | 3: the self-inflicted death of a patient induced by the medication they are prescribed | 4: the cause of such a death by negligence of the prescriber

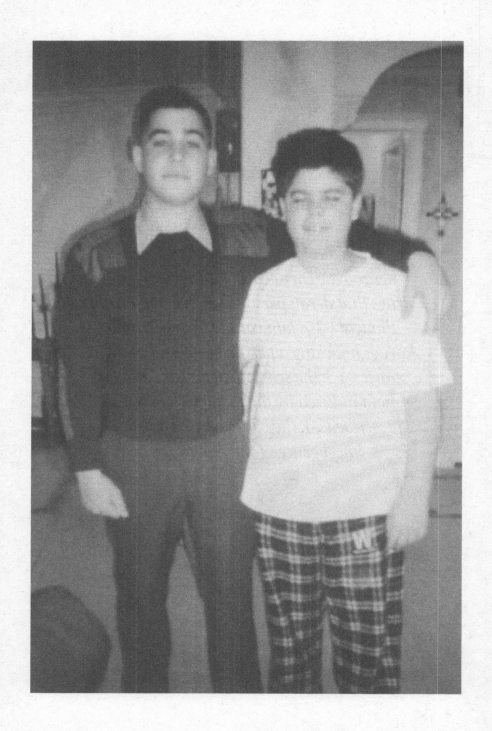

Dedication

This book is dedicated to my beloved sons:
Janos V Lutz and Justin Janos Lutz.

*This book was written for every single veteran that
has passed, is isolating, peeking out from behind their
curtains, and thinking that their lives are over.*

*This book is for every veteran incarcerated because
prescribed pharmaceuticals took control of their minds.*

*It is my hope and prayer that the protocol to treat
our veterans will change to a more holistic, human
approach, and that dangerous pharmaceuticals
will be the last resort.*

Together we will.

Mama Lutz | August 2021

DISCLAIMER

The publisher and author make no representations or warranties of any kind with respect to this book or its contents. The publisher and the author disclaim all such representations and warranties, including but not limited to warranties of healthcare for a particular purpose. Because of the dynamic nature of information and the internet, the publisher and author assume no responsibility for errors, inaccuracies, omissions, or any other inconsistencies herein.

Additionally, the publisher and author make no guarantees concerning the level of success one may experience by following the advice and strategies contained in this book, and the reader understands that he or she accepts the risk that results will differ for each individual. The testimonials, examples, and illustrations provided in this book show results which may not apply to the average reader and are not intended to represent or guarantee that one will achieve the same or similar results.

The content of this book is for informational purposes only and is not intended to diagnose, treat, cure, or prevent any service-connected condition or disease. This book is not intended as a substitute for consultation with a licensed practitioner, VA or otherwise. Please consult with a physician or healthcare specialist regarding the suggestions and recommendations made in this book. The use of any information in this book implies your acceptance of this disclaimer.

Because of the dynamic nature of the Internet, any web addresses or links contained in this book may have changed since publication and may no longer be valid.

TABLE OF CONTENTS

Introduction   *i*

1| THE LAST GOOD DAY   *1*

Let's Take a Drive
Everything Changes
Dishonest Drugs

2| ZOMBIE DOPE   25

Hard Homecoming
Benzos
Opioids
The Benzo Battle

3| THANK YOU FOR YOUR SERVICE   51

Side Effect: Suicide
Almost the Last Day
The Alarming Rate
Bad PR

4| Lonely Days, Lonely Nights — 75

Rizzo's Gift
War and Peace
The Spartan Pledge

5| In the Dark — 101

Who Are You?
HIPAA Hell
TBIs, or the NFL with Guns
Signs of Suicide Ideation

6| Broken Tools — 131

PsyOp
Transitioning Home
Continuing Mission
A Way Forward

7| Living to Tell — 159

Breath and Body
Trauma-Conscious Yoga
What Is Elohim's Breath?
The Way to the Gym
Move It or Lose It

Warfighter Culture
Walking Wounded
You Are What You Eat
Plants, not Poisons
For Good Sleep
On to the Herbs!
For a Brighter Mood
For a Calmer Mind
For Pain Relief
Cannabis

8| LIVE TO TELL   *211*

Breath and Body
Trauma-Conscious Yoga
What Is Elohim's Breath?

Epilogue   *217*
Addendum 1: Aftermath of War   *228*
Addendum 2: The Plan   *232*
Photo Gallery   *234*
Endnotes   *240*
Resources   *251*
About the Author   *253*

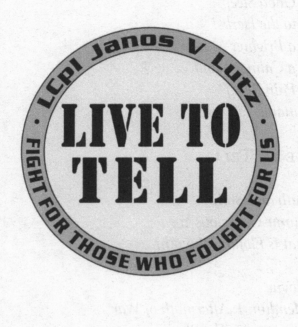

LCpl Janos V Lutz

LIVE TO TELL

· FIGHT FOR THOSE WHO FOUGHT FOR US ·

INTRODUCTION
LIVE TO TELL?

I am Janine Lutz, a Marine mom who fights for those that fought for us. I have a story to tell you about my son John. John was a triple threat, as he was told a few times by the ladies. He was good looking, had big feet, and made the girls swoon when he was in his dress blues.

When John walked into a room, he lit it up with his love of life and wicked sense of humor, yet all the while he was aware of everyone in the room. If there was some-one in need, John would meet those needs. If someone needed a ride, a couple of bucks, or the shirt off his back, John would happily oblige.

I remember one day after Johnny came home from the Marines. We were coming back on I-95 after a day of kay-aking when we came upon an automobile accident. The car was upside down. John said, "Pull over, Mom." I did.

John ran across five lanes of traffic to offer assistance. The car was surrounded by about a dozen people that were rocking the car in an effort to get it right side up with no concern for the injured, unconscious driver. John arrived at the scene, assessed the situation, and took total control. He had the people stop what they were doing, and he scrunched down. Walking on the ceiling of the vehicle on broken glass in bare feet, John cut the seatbelt, lifted the unconscious man, and cautiously laid him on the ground. The ambulance, which had just arrived, was quickly able to attend to this man's injuries. "Wow!" I thought to myself as I beamed with pride. "My Marine son is quite a man."

I recall another time when a school bus stopped in front of our business. John was probably 14 years old then, and being the curious kid that he was, he hurried over to it to see what was up. He discovered that the bus was on fire. He ran into our warehouse, grabbed a fire extinguisher, ran back over to the bus, and extinguished the fire. When he finished helping yet another stranger, he smiled from ear to ear. Nothing made his heart smile more than helping others.

John loved the outdoors and all the creatures in it that he discovered. When John was about 7 years old, we were having an addition built on to our home. Through the open plastic sheeting, a baby possum got into the house. I woke up around midnight when I heard strange noises under a playpen that was in our bedroom. John's dad and I jumped out of bed to realize that a possum was in our bedroom. John's dad screamed, no lie, like a girl. I laughed hysterically, as I did not previously know of his fear of possums.

We called animal control and ended up with a few members of the Davie PD in our home trying to catch this wild animal. The Davie PD tried to no avail. Then my two boys woke to the commotion and came to see what all the fuss was about. We told them what was going on, and John casually replied, "I'll get it." And just like that, John got a towel, cornered the baby possum, threw the towel over it, and picked it up. Again John's dad ran screaming. It was hilarious to see this little boy run after his dad with a baby possum in a towel. I still laugh out loud thinking about that day.

My son John had no fear of anything in nature. He loved everything from spiders and snakes to the great white shark. Growing up, he had a royal python, a tarantula, and a pet rat. Our TV watching was mostly *Animal Planet*, and we looked forward to our yearly dose of *Shark Week*. John loved being outside. He was always off on an adventure on his bicycle, soon to return with an animal that he had caught. He enjoyed the reaction from Mom and Dad when he would walk into the house with his prize.

There are so many wonderful childhood stories to write about. John was fearless, confident, and completely independent ever since he was a toddler. Without a doubt or hesitation, when John made up his mind about something, he did it.

So when John told me he wanted to join the United States Marine Corps, I knew that he was already going to do it, no matter what I said or did to convince him otherwise. I look at his dress blues picture and see my grown son, and I couldn't be a prouder Marine Mom. Not only was my son a United States Marine, but most importantly, he also had a heart for his fellow man. What mother wouldn't be proud of that alone? No—I couldn't possibly be prouder of my boy.

But now my beautiful son isn't tracking sand into my living room anymore, or playing video games in the next room, or taking his dog Kobe for a walk. He's not off at a party with his tight group of high school friends or out shooting with his brother. He's not going to answer a phone call or a text. My son is gone.

No bullet got him. No IED exploded too close. He was a casualty of friendly fire—the kind of fire delivered by a prescription pad. You may not have heard of the term pharmaceutical induced suicide, so I'll give you the rundown on it.

Some of our soldiers come home from war already addicted to the kind of medication that tears at their brains, injecting thoughts and ideas that don't belong to them, that have nothing to do with the kind of people they truly are. Some of them were ordered to take this medication by the VA to deal with symptoms of Post-Traumatic Stress. Instead of naturally processing the horrors they experienced on the battlefield and dealing with all the emotions that arise in them, they get prescribed the zombie dope that leaves them barely alive. When they check out, they're not the ones doing the checking.

The dope pushing is a sick answer to a timeless problem. People have always gone to war since we were cavemen; this is true. But society used to know how to help its warriors through community, faith, and natural practices without medically incapacitating them. And it's only recently that the people who go to war have to fight harder than ever for their very lives once they get back home. And not all of them make it.

Listen, I'm not going to stand on a soap box and scream at you to burn down the VA. Sure, I think they could do a lot of things better, and I hope they do. I'll tell you about some of them later.

What I really want to tell you, if you love a Warfighter like I do, is to pay attention to the details. Learn to read their body language. Remember that your Warfighter is trained to follow orders. They are told to do something and do it without concern for their very lives. This is a very important factor to realize when they are ready to connect with their local Veterans' Administration.

Most importantly, you have to get them in contact with other Warfighters around them. Their brothers and sisters in arms can see things you can't. They can understand things you can't. So open your arms to them, and do all you can to connect with your family of warriors.

There are things I wish I'd known that I just didn't know. There are things I wish I had the chance to do that I just didn't. However, I'm not going to live on the island of the day before and mourn my son forever. I love my son too much to do that.

So, here's what I'm going to do, if you'll come with me. I'm going to tell you straight up what your Warfighter won't about what it's like for them. I'm going to tell you how to pay attention to your Warfighter and when to act. I'm going to enlist your help to make sure that your Warfighter, and all the other Warfighters out there, are safer when they come home, not less safe. With your help, I'm going to make sure that every last one of them will Live to Tell their stories. Just like I'm here to tell mine.

Let me assure you, walking through the death of your kid is no joke. You can't get through it just because you're naturally strong or because you've got good friends looking out for you or because people are sending you thoughts and prayers. Staying alive is sometimes a matter of sheer will, clawing yourself up for the next breath and the next one and the one after that.

By the end of 2016, I was done clawing. I was done trying. I had lost everything I cared about, and I could see no reason to keep going. And I was in a bad way—drinking every night to be numb and eating to die instead of eating to live. So I decided that I was done. I got all my affairs in order so that I could die.

One thing saved me, and I know now that it was a thought that came not from me but from Elohim. I was a pretty logical person, and I knew that I was making this decision out of a bad place. I was also in a lot of physical pain from a bad back. So, I decided to go to a health center, dry out from all the alcohol and caffeine and toxins, get some relief from my pain, and then see what happened with a clear head.

I got my body clean. I did some journaling. I wrote a letter that was powerful and emotional for me and my group. But my back still killed me, and I hadn't changed my mind.

Then my group did some guided breathing together

in a yurt—this circular tent with a wooden frame. It was called transformational breathing, where you breathed deep into your belly. And we all laid with our feet pointed to the middle of this circle. We just started breathing, and I would hear people just suddenly start to cry.

"What the heck is going on here?" I thought. Nothing was happening for me. I felt nothing different. But I made up my mind: "I'm just going to keep breathing." So I just kept breathing. And I was hearing people experiencing different things, making different sounds. But nothing was happening to me. I just continued.

And then all of a sudden, my back spasmed! And everything just came out. I started sobbing. My grief that I had tried to numb and stuff down and ignore so that I could keep going—that grief was released. I was holding it in my back, and it just came out. I had an emotional discharge, and since that day, I have never had a problem with my back again. Isn't that something?

Transformational breathing, which I now call Elohim's breath, was a vital piece of my healing. That and other natural modalities helped me find a way to live. Honoring my son and working with veterans gave me a purpose.

During 2020, when the whole world was going crazy and cringing in fear of the very air around them, I found myself back in a dark place. But it wasn't until the beginning of 2021, when America came to a breaking point, that I found faith, and that faith sparked a life in my soul that I had not felt in a long time. As I could never have imagined feeling again, my heart overflowed with joy and peace. To someone who has already walked through the valley of the shadow of death, never expecting to see the green meadows on the other side, this reawakening was totally unexpected, totally overwhelming, and totally beautiful. When I least expected it, my loving Father handed me relief and peace and a way forward.

That same thing can happen for your loved ones. If they can just keep going, just keep talking, just hang on for the thing that will happen for them, then they can heal. They can Live to Tell their own stories. Though they may not be able to imagine life, hope, purpose, and happiness on the other side of their own Death Valley, you can help them move forward long enough to find them.

I'm organizing this book along the themes of six different qualities that we need to embrace in our mission to stop veteran suicide: Honesty, Independence, Respect, Knowledge, Vision, and Community. I believe that these qualities hold the key to helping us all understand and tackle this tragedy. Afterwards, I will discuss the importance of Faith as an additional virtue that has begun transforming my life.

If we approach veteran suicide from the perspective of these virtues, then Together We Will make a difference for our veteran family. We have to do all we can to make sure that they can all Live to Tell the stories of their lives.

And because Johnny isn't here to tell you his, I will.

MAMA LUTZ | *August 2021*

1

The Last Good Day

MOST people who know me call me Mama Lutz.

Maybe it's because I'm 36% Sicilian according to my DNA testing, but family is one of the most important things to me. If I meet you and I like you, you're part of the family. As the founder of the Lutz Live to Tell Foundation and Lutz Buddy Up Social Clubs that is its flagship program, I'm meeting a lot of young Warfighters, men and women around Johnny's age.

I think they can sense a good mother energy in what I'm trying to do. I'm creating life and building community in places it wasn't obvious before, and I'm fostering life in places where it's in trouble. That kind of devotion to life and the importance of community is what I'm all about.

And I love these veterans. They mean the world to me.

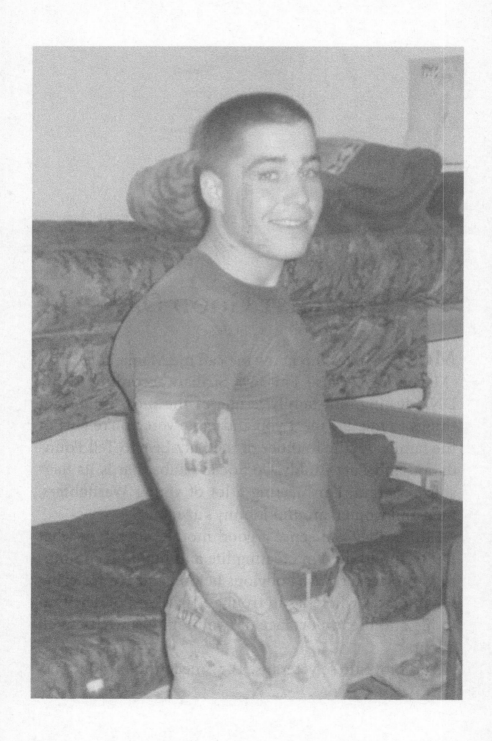

I see them for who they are, and I see them for who they can be. Wherever they are, I'll take em, lumps and all.

It's what I learned to do in the twenty-four years I was lucky enough to be with my son.

And that devotion to life is one reason that I'm going to tell Johnny's story a little differently than you may expect. You're probably expecting me to start with baby stories and pull you forward to the tearful goodbye. Well, I'm not going to do that. We're starting with the last day.

And the reason I want to do that is so that you'll stay with me. I don't want you seeing every event of Johnny's life through this sad filter of "When is it going to happen? How is it going to happen?" No. Let's look at the worst first, and then you can stay with me while we talk about why. And then you can enjoy the stories I'm going to tell you about my kid—because he was a great kid.

So here is the story of the last good day.

"Let's Take a Drive"

Johnny had been a mainly silent presence in our house for a few weeks. Things had gone wrong for him lately. His dog was sick. His girl was gone. I thought he was just moping, understandably and deservedly, but a few weeks after Christmas, I thought it was time he got up, shook the funk off, and did something fun.

"Hey, the weather's nice," I hinted. "How about we cruise in the Maserati?"

The day was a nice and sunny Saturday.

I am blessed to run the family business, like I have for years, and I work hard, as I have most of my life. When I have a day off work, I like to go fast.

Johnny agreed to go out. That was a good sign for me after so much distance and silence. I felt happy to be with him and proud to be seen with him, too. I may have mentioned that he was a handsome guy, and I enjoyed just being with him.

I knew just what to do to make Johnny smile and come back to himself: take him to Executive Airport. Johnny was getting his pilot's license, and the airport was a place where he could touch base with good things about himself and look forward to something he enjoyed.

I drove Johnny to the airport with the convertible top down to enjoy the sun and the wind. First, we browsed the airport store and got some flight merch. Johnny loved the sunglasses there. Then he went to the flight simulator and flew in there for a while.

I sat for a while looking at him with his full beard, well-groomed and so grown up. He had his father's eyes with these long, black eyelashes. My heart just swelled in my chest with pride for this growing man who had survived so much and been so strong.

I wanted to take a picture of him concentrating on the simulator controls so that I could just freeze that moment for myself. No premonition here—just appreciation for where I was and who I was with. Because I didn't want to be the stereotypical pain-in-the-ass mom, I let that moment go. I contented myself with thinking, "Oh, my God! He's so handsome! You know? My son's just so handsome, and he's a Marine!"

*Here is my first gift of knowledge for you. When a human life senses the end approaching, it accepts one last surge of energy. Maybe you've seen this happen with an aging grandparent or a friend who's terminally ill. One day they're lying in bed unable to move, and the next they're up baking a cake or watching the game like nothing's wrong. After that comes the end.

This happens with suicidal people, too.

What I didn't know on that last day was that Johnny hadn't been moping in an ordinary way these last few weeks. He was seriously on the edge of a deep pool of very bad thoughts, and any stray breath could blow him inside and sink him deep. I didn't understand that agreeing to go with me to one of his favorite places was a last gift to me. It was a last reach for the light before the darkness pulled him under.

I just didn't know. Part of me wishes I could go back to that moment staring at my handsome, grown son in that flight simulator and warn myself to put him back in the car and drive him straight to the hospital. I want to scream myself awake and aware. The rest of me knows that that can't happen and that I have to be okay with what I didn't know then. When the regret gets very bad, Yahweh comforts me. But now you know. So pay attention.

When Johnny finished with the flight simulator, we went to this really cool restaurant at the Fort Lauderdale Executive restaurant: Jet Runway. The inside is bright and modern, with light wood floors and sleek white chairs. One whole wall is a window overlooking the runway, where you can see planes take off and land while you eat and chat. Small palms wave in a planter right outside, and beyond the runway, Florida wilderness grows thick and green no matter the time of year.

Johnny and I sat by the window. But instead of watching the planes, Johnny set his chair with his back to the window. "Come on over and sit by me so you can see the planes," I told him.

He shook his head and sat down. "No, Mom, I'm okay."

"Come on," I coaxed, nodding to the view outside. Sunshine and happiness. But he wouldn't budge.

If you love a Warfighter enough to read my son's story, you probably know what was going on. I had a clue about this one. People who have been in combat or in high-stress situations like prisons never sit with their backs exposed to the room. They never give anyone the chance to sneak up behind them. That's what Johnny was doing when he sat down.

Even though I knew that Johnny was only acting according to his training, I was a little disappointed. I had chosen this place especially to give Johnny a little bit of joy. But I set that aside so that I could enjoy time with my son.

He kept his sunglasses on while we waited for our order. I persuaded him to take them off finally, and when he did, I couldn't help but notice how one eyeball seemed jumpy. One was fine, looking straight at me or the table or the room. But the other one panicked back and forth like the pendulum of the world's smallest clock counting down.

"Johnny!" I yelped. "What's wrong with your eye?"

I thought he might have been doing a trick. That would have been like him, like his old self. A good sign. He could stick a nail up his nose! And he knew no limits when it came to pulling off a joke, being the life of the party. The kid would do almost anything for a laugh.

But he wasn't going for a laugh. He wasn't doing anything with his eye. "I don't know," he shrugged.

Neither did I.

*Here's my second gift to you. That particular eyeball motion is a sign that the person is taking Klonopin, a benzodiazepine that is prescribed to treat depression. It's in the same family of drugs as Valium and Ativan, though Klonopin acts differently than other benzos. One of the known side effects of Klonopin is suicide ideation. That drug centers your thoughts on death, whispers death into your ear on a constant loop, leads you to the side of that dark, dark pool and tells you to slip inside.

You understand—the patient using this drug in his own heart and soul and mind does not want to die. The drugs tell him he wants that. The drugs whisper so loud that the patient can't hear hope and life and options and reason. The drugs medically cause the person's death, no matter the instrument of death. That's incidental. The real killer is the benzos.

If I had known how to read that signal, again, we would have been out of those chairs and on our way to the emergency room. But I didn't know. You do. Pay attention.

When the food came, Johnny picked at it. He didn't really eat much of anything, even though the food at Jet Runway is fantastic. At this point, although grateful for a day out with my boy, I was considering the trip to the airport kind of a bust as far as waking Johnny up to himself. Maybe he needed some rest.

We left the restaurant and got in the car to go home.

"Mom," Johnny asked, "can we go to the mall so I can spend those gift cards from Christmas?"

Those gift cards had been lying on the pool table in our home for weeks. The fact that my well-groomed, sharp-dressing son didn't want to get new clothes had been a concern. But I had other plans that night.

"Can't, sorry, I've got a hair appointment for tonight." I was going with a friend to see the Long Island Medium; I was also happy for the chance to dress up and have a girls' night. "But hey, go with your brother. Justin would love to go out with you."

Justin, Johnny's younger brother, adored him. Johnny, the older brother, the daring brother, the popular brother, the combat-hardened Marine, was Justin's hero and always had been. I shouldn't hoard the wealth now that Johnny was up and moving around. I should let Justin have some brother time.

"Okay," Johnny agreed.

I was happy. Any mommas out there know that watching your kids get along is a real heart-warmer.

Johnny then asked me if a particular store in the mall was still open (I forget which), as he hadn't been there in a while and he had a gift card for it.

"I don't know; Google it," I told him. He said he would.

I was so happy to see him planning a night out for himself and his brother, reaching for a good thing, a little happiness. I took it as a good sign. I thought he was on his way back to himself.

After I dropped Johnny off at the house, I went to my hair appointment. When I got back home to get dressed for the show, the boys were gone to the mall, and the gift cards were gone from the pool table, at long last. Johnny was Carpe-ing the hell out of this Diem for the first time in a while. I got into my car with a light heart and picked up my girlfriend for the show.

I don't know if you've ever had the pleasure of seeing the Long Island Medium, Theresa Caputo. She's a priceless mix of *Jersey Shore* and *The Sixth Sense*. Her show did not disappoint. I mean, how can talking to people on the other side ever be boring?

Before the show started, at about 7 o'clock, Johnny

called me.

"Mom, are you home?"

"No, honey, I told you I was going to the show. Why, what's up?"

"Oh, I got a flat tire," he explained. He did long-distance bike riding, so the flat tire sounded plausible to me.

The man I was dating at the time was available to help if Johnny needed, so I suggested that Johnny call him.

"He'll come get you."

"Oh, no, that's okay. I'll just handle it."

That was the old Johnny—thoughtful and independent. Capable and calm. Outside, like he loved to be.

But he was lying to me. It was the last time I ever heard his voice.

I put my phone on silent, sat back beside Paulette, and relaxed. If you were wondering, here is where things got super bad. Just a fair warning.

But before they get bad, I want to tell you something, if you love a Warfighter. There is nothing wrong with going out and enjoying yourself, even if something bad happens while you do. You are a human being, and you can't be in full-on attention mode every second of every day and night when you're around someone who needs help. If you try to be, you'll end up worn-out and depressed yourself.

No matter what responsibilities you have with your Warfighter, you have to take care of yourself. You have to enjoy the world and let yourself relax. You are not some heroic sacrifice on the altar of patriotism or family. You are a person.

Enjoy being a person.

"Everything Changes"

Theresa's show that night was great. I had a wonderful time, and when it was over at around 10:30, I picked up my phone to check my messages in my seat while the crowd began to filter out.

My younger son Justin had called me three times.

That was not normal for Justin, who was a pretty self-sufficient young man and not a big talker. Slightly concerned, I dialed him back.

"Hey, honey," I began.

He cut me off. "Why don't you answer your fucking phone? Johnny's dead. Get home."

And then the world stopped.

I don't have any memory of what I said or did next.

Justin hung up on me.

Nothing was real.

I only realized that I was panicking when other people around me started to gather and show concern. But they weren't concerned enough for anything to be real.

If my tall, handsome, laughing boy was really gone, why wasn't the place on fire?

Why weren't people screaming at the top of their lungs, running around and shaking each other?

Why weren't people collapsing to the floor in shock?

This was big fucking news. What was wrong with everybody?

Finally, I said something to Paulette, and she said, "What! Who called you? Give me your phone!" She took my phone and called back. The man I was seeing at the time answered. Paulette handed me the phone, and he said to me, "Johnny's dead."

Looking back on that night, I can't help but think, "How do you just say that to somebody?" Don't you give them some preface? Like, "Are you sitting down?" or "Can you come home?" Or don't even tell the person. Just get them home, right?

Because I couldn't even function after that. I couldn't even get out of the chair. I actually became part of that chair. I didn't even want to face what I had to face. I had tunnel vision, and everything was foggy and surreal.

And then I started getting louder.

"What am I going to do? No—I can't—this can't be!" It was something like that. I was in shock. I don't remember what I was saying.

And then I called my nephew Chris.

"Chris, Johnny's dead, Chris! What am I going to do! Chris, Chris!"

He had heard. Justin had called him when he couldn't reach me. He'd called his father, too, and his father had come to him. I didn't know that until later, of course.

During the call with Chris, I just still sat there. I had

no idea how long I sat. It might have been five minutes. It might have been twenty. I don't know.

By this time, the police came to me because the place was clearing out. Some lady behind me had her hand on my shoulder. I was grieving, obviously. The irony was that the Long Island Medium had just been talking to dead people, right? So people were thinking that I was freaking out because I was talking to somebody dead—long dead.

You can't make this shit up.

A police officer asked Paulette, "What's going on here?"

"Her son died," Paulette explained.

"All right, when did her son die?"

Paulette must have said, "Just now," or something like that, because the policeman said, "Who's she talking to? Can I talk to who she's talking to?" He took the phone, and Chris, who was still on the other line said, "Her son just died."

Then I got it in me. The news gelled into something close to reality. I didn't fully accept it, but I could move and speak and think a little. I looked at Paulette and the police officers and said, "I've got to get home to my boy. I need to get home and see my boy."

Paulette and I got up and walked to the car. I couldn't drive; so Paulette drove. When we got home, however, we couldn't even get on the property and had to stay across the street. Johnny's death was a crime scene, and you couldn't enter. You couldn't be there unless you'd been there all along. I hadn't.

I only found out what happened later.

After I dropped Johnny off at home that afternoon, Johnny and Justin went shopping. Johnny must have bought around $300 worth of clothes with his Christmas gift cards. When they were finished shopping, both of my boys went to their dad's apartment, which was right around the corner. And no, that had never been weird for me. I may have been divorced, but I still cared about the father of my kids. I wanted him to see his boys as often as he could. Living close was convenient.

Their dad cooked them a barbecue with burgers. And just like at the airport restaurant, Johnny didn't eat. He left early, leaving Justin behind, because he wanted to come home alone. The drugs inside him were driving him to his end, but there was enough of Johnny left in charge that he wanted to protect his little brother that way.

Just like he had tried to protect me. Remember when Johnny called me about the flat tire before the show? He was checking to see where I was to make sure that I wasn't going to be home before he finished.

When Johnny got home, he sat down at his computer and wrote a note to me and Justin and his father. He apologized for causing us pain, but he was going to be out of pain. Finally.

He took a black marker and wrote on his door DNR: *Do not resuscitate.* He wrote the same thing on his forehead.

The drugs in his brain did not want him coming back up from that dark pool they'd been luring him to enter.

Then my son checked out.

No, I'm not going to tell you how. Some people in a dark place use those kinds of details for an instruction manual, and I'm not going to give that to anybody. The fact that he is gone is enough.

When Justin got home from his father's place, he went down the hall to find his brother. Instead, Justin found the note on Johnny's door. No brother should ever have to see what Justin did. Johnny's body was already cold.

Justin kept the depth of the hell he went through to himself. Later, he told me details when I asked, but he could never fully explain the torture of that sight, the way it ripped his heart into pieces. How could he? So that was his burden to carry.

My boyfriend was already at home when Justin found Johnny. Justin probably yelled for him or went and got him. I don't know if Justin called me first or if he called 911 first or his father. When his father found out, he came rushing over to my house and made my boyfriend leave. Even though my boyfriend lived with me, that's how Johnny's father was. His boy was dead. His other boy was in trouble. I wasn't there. Therefore, he was in charge.

My boyfriend obliged because of the situation. He waited across the street on the neighbor's lawn for me to come home. Justin called my nephew Chris and told him what had happened.

15

The paramedics came. They did what they were required to do, but they were working on a cold body. There was no way to revive him. They all knew it.

Then the police came, locked down the scene, and started investigating.

But they were investigating the wrong place.

They should have been investigating the makers of Klonopin, the VA doctors that prescribed it knowing full well that it causes suicidal ideations, and the government bureaucrats that decided on the opioid and benzo regimen instead of alternate therapies that help. That work. That's where the police should have been locking things down.

I came home to a cold night on the neighbor's front lawn, waiting to do something, anything. I can't describe to you how I felt on that night of purgatory—not in the world where Johnny no longer existed and not yet in the house where he no longer lived. I wish I had known at the time how close Elohim was to me. I wish I had been able to feel that love and peace at the moment I needed it most.

But I was lost, and I felt alone and confused. My brain ran a loop of anger and grief and regret and numbness with no order and no hope of stopping until the police emerged and let me in.

When they finally did, I wanted to see Johnny. The detective doing the investigation advised against it.

"Well, you can see him if you want to, but I'm telling

you to keep the memory in your head of your son that you spent time with today."

I said, "Okay." That's what I did.

You may feel differently. You may have needed to see the body to prove that the worst had happened. I didn't. I had that mental picture of my beautiful, strong Marine concentrating on that flight simulator with the Florida sun touching his hair and his cheeks and his beautiful blue eyes that very afternoon. That was the picture I wanted to keep.

The following days passed in a blur. People came and went. I remember some of the ones who showed up. Danielle, Johnny's friend from high school, came and sat with me and had dinner most nights in the beginning. Kevin Ullman, Johnny's former roommate, came the day after Johnny died to take care of everything from the funeral arrangements to cleaning out Johnny's car and his room. My nephew Chris Hayes came the same day to make sure Justin and I were okay and to take care of anything that we needed. Joe and Kevin dressed John in his dress blues.

We had a funeral, open casket so that everyone could see Johnny's face one last time. It was his face, but it wasn't him. You could tell that the real Johnny was somewhere far, far away, somewhere I don't think even the Long Island Medium could ever find him.

In addition to the people who had come immediately to help, other people attended the funeral. Johnny's high school friends arrived, stunned and grieving. Nick Rizzo from the 2/8 Marines came, along with others from the regiment.

The Marines who had served with Johnny performed a roll call and walked up to the casket. To see Johnny's band of brothers around him touched me deeply, along with everyone else in the room. Last, the Marines called Johnny's name. No reply. There never would be again. And when I came home again and there was nothing else to do, nothing else to organize or decide, the loss hit me in a whole new way.

I was lost without Johnny.

I couldn't even begin to know how to deal with that kind of grief and pain on a daily basis. I felt as if a heavy blanket had been thrown over me, cutting off the air and light and sound of the normal world and stifling me in alternating waves of numbness and pain.

I spent five months under that blanket. I couldn't find a way out of it.

Then one day, for no reason I could tell you, I woke up mad.

Anger is good for me. It clarifies my thoughts so that I can listen to my gut. And my gut told me that I needed to find out what happened to my son.

Here is what I found.

"Dishonest Drugs"

We'll start with a really dishonest drug policy in relation to our Warfighters. It has its roots in some pretty far-out places, but the effects today are all too real. Some problems our veterans are facing are directly due to a lack of honesty in our federal government.

In 1953, the CIA began systematic research into creating a Manchurian candidate-type super soldier: someone who was programmed for unquestioning obedience. Americans were fairly certain that Russians were already engaged in this type of research to be used against our service members.[1] During Operation Paperclip, former Nazi scientists informed our government about a Swiss drug that could incapacitate enemy personnel without killing them. That drug was LSD, and the research into using it to create a super soldier occurred under Operation Bluebird, otherwise known as MK Ultra.[2]

To create this soldier, CIA agents dosed unsuspecting people (including soldiers) with LSD, ecstasy, heroin, mushrooms, and other drugs, and then watched and recorded the results. The fallout from this research got so bad that President Gerald Ford was forced to issue an apology and to sign an executive order banning "experimentation with drugs on human subjects, except with the informed consent, in writing and witnessed by a disinterested party, of each such human subject."[3]

Of course, by then the search for the super soldier was on, and research existed to prove that drugs could alter someone's personality and decision-making. But the research proved that most drugs they had already tested didn't make someone compliant. Instead, they made people stop thinking logically and lose their inhibitions.

So the military began capitalizing on that aspect of a new drug used for a reasonable task: preventing malaria. Giving someone a new drug for a supposedly good reason wasn't human testing, really. It was just using a new drug. That drug, which now carries a black-box warning of its dangerous side effects, was mefloquine.[4]

Mefloquine was first developed by researchers at Walter Reed. As far back as 1983, the World Health Organization was calling Mefloquine "by no means ideal" and recording harmful psychological and physical side effects. However, there was no other drug available to combat resistant strains of malaria being found in Southeast Asia.[5]

Our government gave the patent for Mefloquine to Roche, a Swiss chemicals and pharmaceuticals company which also manufactured the lion's share of benzodiazepines like Valium and Klonopin. Pretty generous gift, huh? It has made Roche millions over the years since 1982.[6]

Mefloquine is also sold retail under the brand name Lariam, and travelers to malaria-prone areas, such as Peace Corps volunteers, also take it and have reported some of the same side effects. Theirs do not appear as severe as those reported by military service members for the simple reasons that 1) they are free to stop taking Lariam when they notice side effects and 2) their minds are not stocked with images and sounds of the trauma of war. Common sense tells anyone that a college kid will hallucinate different dangers than a combat vet.

Despite the fact that Mefloquine should be taken between a week and two weeks before exposure to malaria risk, our Warfighters receive their first dose of Mefloquine as they are getting on the plane to deploy. They take it regularly in country, once per week—some joke about "Mefloquine Mondays." And these doses do not appear in their medical charts.[7] Now I ask you, if the government was being above-board and honest about administering these pills to prevent malaria, why wouldn't the dose appear in the medical charts?

The reason is that some of the dangerous side effects of Mefloquine work to the advantage of a government that wants more effective Warfighters. Are they unthinking, programmable shells, like the CIA initially wanted? No. But they are more reckless. The self-preservation instinct in their brains turns off. So they'll act first, without considering whether they'll survive. If I was sending a young man into the teeth of gunfire, I'd certainly want that side effect, as much of it as I could get.[8]

However, the men who show signs of Mefloquine toxicity seldom get a correct diagnosis. Why is that? In order to diagnose anyone with Mefloquine toxicity, a psychiatrist has to rule out 1) exposure to other drugs 2) pre-existing mental conditions 3) poor record-keeping of Mefloquine exposure or 4) use of alcohol or other psychotropic drugs.

If you love someone in the military, let me ask you: what veteran do you know personally that 1) hasn't taken any other prescribed drugs that may have induced the same side effects 2) doesn't have PTS or TBI 3) has perfect records of every Mefloquine taken while in the service 4) never drinks or experiments with drugs? Even venerable old Korean War vets who are pure as the driven snow have surely taken other prescribed medications and/or had a TBI during service. [9]

Take for instance the case of Bill Manofsky. Bill served in Iraq and Kuwait as part of the Gulf War.[10] A commanding officer handed him foil packs of Mefloquine to take for malaria prevention, and Bill took them. Soon he began having symptoms that included sensitivity to light, vertigo, hallucinations, and tremors. Civilian doctors back in the States diagnosed Mefloquine toxicity and began treating him, even though the Navy questioned the diagnosis and put him through a full medical board to make sure that he wasn't "malingering."[11]

But Bill wasn't malingering. He had suffered a permanent brain injury from taking that drug—to prevent malaria. In the desert. Where there are no mosquitos. Though it went against common sense, Bill explained that contracting an illness or a condition like malaria or sunburn could get you in trouble for dereliction of duty, especially if you'd been given a preventative like Mefloquine or sunscreen. Bill notes that there is no practical, medical reason for anyone to take malaria prophylaxis in the desert or high in the mountains of Afghanistan.[12]

Bill consulted a prominent doctor, Dr. Remington Nevin, epidemiologist, former Army doctor, and expert consultant on antimalaria drugs, particularly Mefloquine. He has written extensively on cases involving Mefloquine toxicity. For years, Dr. Nevin has been writing on the dangers of Mefloquine and other drugs like it, and the depth of his research is truly staggering. He was part of the effort that succeeded in getting that black box warning onto containers of Mefloquine. He's provided expert testimony for people affected by this drug, which he considers terribly dangerous.[13]

So why is our government issuing dangerous drugs that are not necessary for a mission and pressuring Warfighters to take them? It is pretty apparent that despite the Gerald Ford 1976 executive order against human testing of drugs without the subject's consent, the military is doing just that. It's giving a brain-altering, brain damaging drug to our Warfighters purely for the side effects. And that is not acting with honesty.

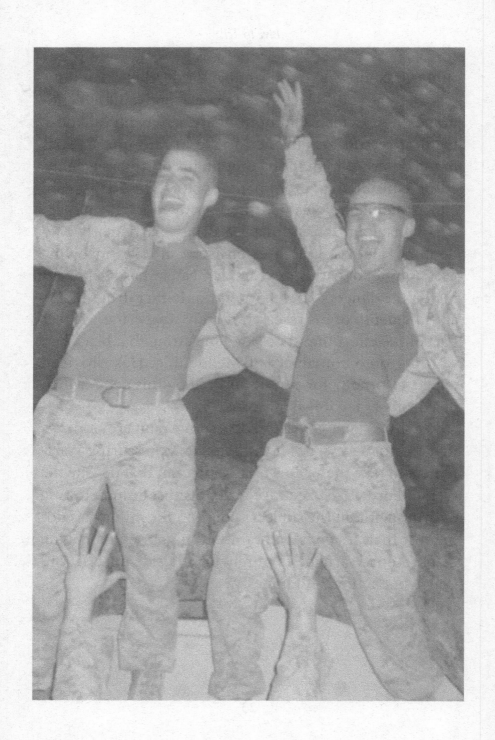

2

ZOMBIE DOPE

JOHNNY'S last day alive was January 12, 2013. Just 8 days before his death, he visited the VA near our home in Sunrise. There, he made decisions that were not in character with the son that I knew. The son that came home from Camp LeJeune was a very different man than the one that went away.

"HARD HOMECOMING"

I wondered about that coming home, how that was for Johnny, and so I talked to one of his friends, Mike Lichtenstein, a JROTC buddy from high school.[14] Mike graduated a year ahead of Johnny and went into the Navy around the same time Johnny went into the Marines. They saw each other from time to time on leaves during the four years they both served. And after his service, Mike came home, too.

But he hadn't intended to come home; that wasn't the plan. After all, Mike went into the Navy partly to be somewhere new and to take advantage of whatever new opportunities came his way. Mike came from a home like ours, one where his parents were amicably divorced—so amicably that Mike jokes they could be British.

Johnny and Mike lived in the same town, went to the same high school, and hung around the same group of friends. Johnny was wilder, more outgoing, the funny one. Mike was steadier, more reserved, the practical one. Mike was practical enough to try college for a while after high school and practical enough to see after a year that it wasn't right for him.

Living at home, managing a pizza place nearby (the same one where he'd worked in high school), and going to school close to home just didn't feel like progress. After sitting in a classroom since kindergarten, Mike was ready to get out and do something. The Navy was a logical path forward. They'd take care of his education, help him become more self-disciplined, and show him the world. Mike was totally on board.

So he went through training and ended up on a submarine, maintaining the engines. The place was really loud, and the life was very isolated. Mike could be underwater for six months at a time, with little news of what was going on in the outside world. The systems he had to maintain were a patchwork of technology bought and installed over time; so Mike got good at troubleshooting problems and coming up with creative solutions. The discipline he knew he needed shaped him day by day.

When he came home on leave and saw Johnny, the boys traded stories and debated who was the real badass. But it wasn't a put-down contest with these boys.

"Look, I always made a distinction between the level of danger I faced and the level Johnny faced," Mike told me. "He would always tell me, 'No, you're the badass,' but nobody was shooting at me. I never went to Iraq or Afghanistan. I'd tell him, 'I have a bed and a shower and air conditioning. You're the badass.'"

It was like Johnny to see the danger his friend was in and acknowledge it. He could be generous that way, because he didn't have a big ego that needed to be fed constantly. He didn't need to one-up his childhood friend to legitimize his own danger.

And it's true: Marines face a different kind of danger. I'm not saying that any work any veteran does isn't important, so nobody out there should get butthurt over that statement. But if you are in the service or service connected, you know that of the four branches, the Army and Marines generally have the most direct contact with the enemy. And the Marines almost always go in first, when things are the worst.

When Mike was mentioning the fact that he had a bed and a shower and air conditioning, he was noting true differences between his service and Johnny's. I'll talk more later about what Johnny's service was like, and why it made a difference in the way Mike left and the way Johnny left. *Because it did.*

After five years of Navy service, Mike got out and transitioned home with high hopes—ones that didn't materialize right away. "My last two years in the Navy, I heard constantly from guys that had some fantastic job lined up. It was something super easy with huge pay, like sitting behind a desk for $145K a year. And some relative was hiring them; so it was a sure thing. But I got out and started working my hardest trying to find a place for myself, and part of me couldn't help thinking, "Where's my big break? Where's my easy job?"

The jobs didn't fall into Mike's lap. He had planned to move near Atlanta, where his fiancée was finishing school and training for her medical career. Surely he could get a job at a fire station or something similar. But the city wouldn't let a guy with speeding tickets near their vehicles.

"That was a real setback for me. I started interviewing for other jobs and found out all the things I didn't have. I didn't have a degree in engineering. I didn't have experience with the latest technology in the field. I didn't have a second language. I learned that in the civilian world, what matters is what piece of paper you can show. You need a degree; you need a certification from your industry. Navy papers don't count. Civilians need certifications."

That was how Mike found himself back at home, back in his childhood bedroom, back at the pizza place, and back at the college he had left five years before. And that was when the anger arrived, a slow burn that flashed out under provocation from time to time.

"Why were you so angry?" I probed. I'd seen those same flashes from Johnny sometimes. I wanted to understand the slow burn that kept them near the surface.

"Some of that anger came from feeling displaced in a way," Mike explained. "It's a weird feeling. One day you're in, and the next day you're out. One day you have a job and a routine and expectations and responsibilities, and then that's all gone. Then what do you do? This was my identity for five years, and then it just wasn't.

"Only it still was for me. When Johnny died, I was out of the Navy, but I still wore my uniform to his funeral. When another of our friends, Andy, died a few months later, I wore my uniform to his funeral, too. I felt inside that I was still part of the military, that this was still my calling. As far as my head and my heart, I might as well have just been on leave."

I could understand that loss of identity. I could understand not having a mission anymore, not being in a situation where your skills and your heart and your physical training were not only wanted but vital. I could see that in Johnny, in his drifting from thing to thing to take up his time without anything lighting the purposeful, sure spark in him that I'd seen when he enlisted.

Mike added, "There's a frustration that comes with not having regimented time and the same kind of life you had before, and that just boiled over. For me, I was right back where I started before I ever went into the military. I couldn't help feeling like I'd gone back in time. Like what was the last five years about? I was stuck in a time warp."

So in addition to the loss of identity, the loss of mission, there was the loss of routine and the lack of visible progress. I could see how Johnny would feel similar. I could walk down the hall to his bedroom, which was just the same way he had left it. Physical ties to his boyhood were everywhere.

I had thought they would be comforting, that he'd like to see his old stuff and feel like he was home. But hearing Mike talk, I could see it another way. Maybe those ties mocked him. Maybe they told him that he hadn't accomplished anything. Maybe they were a stopped clock, a time warp, a quicksand pit of video games and sports trophies that pulled a veil over the time when he was an adult and dangerous and necessary and independent.

But I'd have to ponder that thought later so that I wouldn't miss what Mike was telling me.

"Before I went into the military, I thought that everything would be better when I got out. And it was in some ways. I was more driven with school; I worked harder at it. The military helped me grow up. I'm thankful for the Navy. But when I first got out, I didn't understand what I'd done wrong."

Disappointed expectations. Boy, did Johnny know about those. But that's a story for the next chapter.

"Another thing was that I got home in February," Mike said gently. "John died in mid-January. That was some shit timing. I kept thinking, *If I was home, it wouldn't have happened.*

Yep. Those deaths. The ones you see and the ones you bear. Johnny's heart was full of ghosts. I got that.

I got the guilt, too.

"2013 was a hard year. John and I had another friend, Andy Penta, who was a Marine. He was a good friend. He was sent to Iraq for one tour. He was in a state platoon—not a sniper, but not regular infantry, either. He was working for Academy, which was a subsidiary of Blackwater. He was planning to come home, run his own personal training business, and propose to his girlfriend. He died in May.

"We were all JROTC buddies from high school, most of us class of '05, like me, and John in class of '06. Our friend group went to two funerals in less than five months. And we haven't recovered."

How do you recover from something like that? How do you recover from the massive loss of such young people? Old people we understand. Sick people after a long stretch of pain we can understand, too. But young, healthy Warfighters gone in the blink of an eye—it does something to your soul to bear that loss.

What Mike was describing was a normal, human response to grief and stress. For him, it came out in anger. But Mike wasn't sick. He didn't have head trauma or a psychiatric problem. He was a human person going through a hard time.

"So you're obviously doing better now," I said. "What helped?"

"I did use the VA for anger management when I first got out," Mike said. "I didn't have medical insurance; so the VA was my insurance. My fiancée and my mom really wanted me to go there and get some help. At first I was hesitant. You know, there's a stigma to getting counseling. But it did help. My counselor gave me some coping skills and helped me learn to predict my reactions. I used that. It still helps me. I had a really good experience."

"But you weren't on meds," I pressed. The meds made *all* the difference. I knew that, unfortunately.

"No, I didn't have any meds, and that's because I told them I didn't want any. I wanted to do my treatment without any medication, mostly because of what happened to Johnny. And I knew that I could because of my mom. She has a master's in social work; so I'm familiar with what she does. I told my VA counselor in the first session what happened with John. She respected my decision completely and said, 'Let's get to work.'"

It was bittersweet hearing this affirming story from Mike. For him, the VA worked like it was supposed to. His counselor listened to him and provided only the help he needed, no more. She gave him a useful emotional toolkit for understanding and dealing with his anger.

I wish it had worked that way with Johnny. *Why didn't it?*

For one thing, Mike wasn't injured. He got a minor disability rating for hearing loss that he incurred in those loud engine rooms on the submarines all those years. But he wasn't disabled, and he wasn't in constant physical pain. That's great.

But again, that's because of the different service that Johnny entered. Mike was covering the enemy from the water far away—a necessary and honorable service. No question. But Johnny was kicking in doors, dodging bullets, and getting thrown into a ditch. What my son did was no more or less honorable than any other service out there.

It just fucked up his body in a whole different way. And it led to his being prescribed benzodiazepines.

Benzos

At first, benzodiazepines seemed harmless. Hoffman-LaRoche, a Swiss chemicals company that began in 1896 by making and selling vitamins, employed Leo Sternbach, a brilliant chemist that the company moved from Switzerland to New Jersey in 1941, enabling him to escape the Holocaust.[15] Sternbach, a quiet, kind man who loved his work, stayed with Hoffman-LaRoche, now known simply as Roche, his entire life.[16]

While doing work on dyes for Roche in the 1950s, Sternbach discovered a chemical compound that had muscle-relaxing and calming qualities. Within just a few years, that compound, chlordiazepoxide, had been approved by the FDA. Roche marketed it under the brand name Librium and followed it just a few years later with the most famous benzo: diazepam, also known as Valium.[17]

Benzodiazepines get their name because they connect a ring of benzine with a ring of diazepine. They work because they excite the nervous system to excrete more GABA neurotransmitters.[18] People who don't have enough GABA can suffer from conditions like epilepsy, COPD, and Huntington's disease. So medication that makes sufferers excrete more GABA can soothe tremors and make life bearable.[19]

Excreting more GABA can also chemically soothe feelings of anxiety. However, long-term use of benzos in this way can lead to the opposite effects in the body. Psychiatrist Kelly Brogan details the increase of anxiety, sleeplessness, depression, loss of impulse control, loss of memory, and paranoia as a result of taking benzos. And the withdrawal symptoms are the same but worse—including seizures and suicides. One patient of hers had a grand mal seizure after missing one dose of Xanax.[20]

The *British Journal of General Practice* noted a troubling case history.[21] A 62-year old man who took no other prescriptions and who had no history of mental or psychological problems started taking benzos for sadness after his wife was diagnosed with cancer. His doctor switched him from lorazepam to fluoxetine to alprazolam to temazepam when he began showing anxiety and panic. He also began ordering benzos off the internet. After showing distress at his wife's oncology appointment, he was then given diazepam and Zopiclone. Riddled with anxiety, he ended up stabbing himself in the stomach. When doctors reduced his dosage in an effort to wean him off the benzos, he stabbed himself in the neck and chest.

Warnings against benzos abound. WebMD cautioned that administering Xanax and Valium to patients in a study group with both PTSD and COPD led to twice the suicide rate of those not given the drugs.[22] Texas State University researchers found that prescriptions for benzos led to an increased suicide rate among the elderly.[23] *The Journal of Clinical Psychiatry,* while warning of the suicide risk to those taking benzos, also noted that they are not effective in the treatment of PTSD.[24]

Klonopin is a benzo primarily associated with calming seizures in epileptics, but it can be prescribed for anxiety and panic attacks.[25] Warnings among physicians generally apply to overdose or addiction.[26] The general wisdom among doctors is that the drug is safe unless misused or unless the patient becomes addicted.[27] In fact, Psychiatry Advisor responded to a study on the dangers of opioids and benzos by saying that the dangers were due to misuse.[28] But that is not what patients are finding.

One writer with *USA Today* told the story of his wife's battle with benzo withdrawal. She started taking Klonopin for anxiety and soon experienced pain, insomnia, and diarrhea. After her doctor increased her dosage, she began going into tolerance withdrawal and experiencing a worsening of side effects as well as the original complaint. While she tapered off Klonopin, she endured a hellish bout with an increase of all her symptoms. And though she is now completely free of the drug, her body has not completely healed.[29]

Though the effects of benzos on the body are real, people who report negative side effects to doctors may not get help because of the doctor bias toward the effectiveness of prescription drugs. And that response may leave patients feeling helpless or dismissed.[30] With no help in sight from the people who prescribed these drugs in the first place, no wonder many tormented benzodiazepine patients see suicide as their only relief from constant mental and physical pain.

"Opioids"

Together with opioids, benzos form the basis of the regime of zombie dope that is robbing life from our Warfighters. My dear friend Boone Cutler gave a radio interview in which he shared his own experience with the zombie dope—an experience that nearly led to his death. The opioids prescribed by VA doctors first damaged his kidneys, and then damaged his heart. Suffering from cardiomyopathy, Boone traveled to Panama for stem cell therapy, which saved his life and put him on the path to-wards health.[31]

Another deadly solution the VA is pawning off on our veterans is indefinite reliance on opioids. Nearly every news outlet in America is full of the news of opioid addiction. People overdose continually. Crooked doctors are selling prescriptions to addicts.[32] States are suing manufacturers like Johnson & Johnson[33] (yes, the baby shampoo people) and Purdue[34] (not the chicken people) for the damage to American society that opioids are causing. Yet somehow the VA still views long-term opioid dependence as a valid solution.

The logic escapes me.

Opioids have a far different origin story than benzos do. Ready for this? They all come from the opium poppy. Just like morphine. Just like opium. Just like heroin.[35]

Even if they're not physically made by processing opium poppy flowers like the illegal street drugs, they're artificially concocted to resemble the chemical structure of those little red flowers. And you guys know what those little red flowers do to people, right?

They make you check out. They send you to sleep. Remember Dorothy and the rest in Oz, crossing the field of red flowers and passing out before they can get to the Emerald City? Opium reference. Remember nasty Mrs. Dubose in *To Kill a Mockingbird,* who sat spaced out and drooling while Jem read to her? Opium reference. Remember the Sherlock Holmes story "The Man with the

Twisted Lip" where Watson finds Holmes in an opium den, lost in a mass of people out of their minds?

Yep, our grandparents and great-grandparents knew just what to think of the opium poppy and its derivatives. They gave it to cancer patients with no hope of recovery. They gave it to surgery patients to spare them from feeling their procedures.

They didn't give them to strong, respectable men and women who were feeling sad about real trauma, having trouble sleeping, or feeling long-term physical pain. They knew that opioid dependence was a real and troubling threat. They had enough sense to treat that powerful drug with respect, as a last resort.

We think we know better. We think that if something comes in a little brown bottle from the pharmacy, it's okay. The process of getting a prescription and going to a store counter for a drug whitewashes the stigma for us.

But it doesn't change the nature of the drug.

Most troubling for me is the fact that VA doctors commonly prescribe opioids and benzos together in a cocktail many Warfighters call "zombie dope" for obvious reasons. It's what you take to become a zombie, to sit in a chair while your heart beats and you respirate but to let life slide by you in a fog. And it works as long as you keep breathing. Listen to this.

"Long-term use can cause tolerance, meaning that increased doses are required to achieve the same effect, and physical dependence, meaning that abruptly discontinuing the drug leads to unpleasant withdrawal symptoms. The euphoria attracts recreational use and frequent, escalating recreational use of opioids typically results in addiction. An overdose or concurrent use with other depressant drugs like benzodiazepines commonly results in death from respiratory depression."[36]

Are you serious? It's *common* for opioids and benzos to cause death from respiratory depression—which means that you stop breathing—and it's also *common* for the VA to prescribe these drugs together? Does that make *common* sense to anyone?

And if you don't die on the combination, you can look forward to these lovely side effects from opioid use: "sleep apnea, alcohol use, or kidney problems… Constipation, Drowsiness, Nausea and vomiting."[37] Other side effects can "include itchiness, sedation, nausea, respiratory depression, constipation, and euphoria." And all that is not to mention the sketchy, hard-to-define relationship between opioid use and mental illnesses like depression.[39]

And Warfighters are not the only people who are suffering from this flood of opioids on the medical market. Addiction to opioids is now a national crisis.[40] The statistics nationally are sobering:

"From 1999 to 2017, more than 700,000 people have died from a drug overdose.

Around 68% of the more than 70,200 drug overdose deaths in 2017 involved an opioid.

In 2017, the number of overdose deaths involving opioids (including prescription opioids and illegal opioids like heroin and illicitly manufactured fentanyl) was 6 times higher than in 1999.

On average, 130 Americans die every day from an opioid overdose.

From 1999-2017, almost 400,000 people died from an overdose involving any opioid, including prescription and illicit opioids.

This rise in opioid overdose deaths can be outlined in three distinct waves.

1. The first wave began with increased prescribing of opioids in the 1990s, with overdose deaths involving prescription opioids (natural and semi-synthetic opioids and methadone) increasing since at least 1999.

2. The second wave began in 2010, with rapid increases in overdose deaths involving heroin.

3. The third wave began in 2013, with significant increases in overdose deaths involving synthetic opioids—particularly those involving illicitly-manufactured fentanyl (IMF). The IMF market continues to change, and IMF can be found in combination with heroin, counterfeit pills, and cocaine.[41]

The threat of illegally manufactured drugs is real. Some fentanyl shipped in from China is deadly.[42] But con men are not alone in trying to make a quick buck off the pain of others. The pharmaceutical industry has been doing it for years.

The Sackler family that runs Purdue ramped up marketing of the opioids it manufactures for years after it knew the danger of the drug.[43] According to the *New Yorker Magazine,* "an addiction specialist said that the Sacklers' firm, Purdue Pharma, bears the 'lion's share' of the blame for the opioid crisis."[44] Yet after a bankruptcy filing, which will allow the company to restructure its debt, Purdue will stay in business, keep making and selling more opioids than anyone needs, and keep raking in the money.[45]

Because just like Roche and the manufacturing of benzodiazepines, Purdue and Johnson & Johnson are out for money. Pills are big business, and they're doing a lot of it. And these lawsuits filed by the states to recover some of the damages done to them by a sudden tidal wave of addicts will do only temporary damage to these giant corporations.

Meanwhile, the states will have to keep caring for new additions to the foster care system.[46] Local coroners, police, and prosecutors will have to keep bearing the burden of investigating and dealing with the fallout of wrongful deaths.[47] The young, the troubled, and the poor will have to pay disproportionately in grief and lost life for the profits of the pharmaceutical industry.[48]

Dr. Anna Lembke has a fabulous TED Talk that outlines the causes of the opioid epidemic, along with some possible solutions. She points to the modern medical industry that is substituting pills for personal care, dealing with problems medically that aren't really medical in nature (poverty, homelessness, trauma, abuse), and reinforcing a pain narrative that doesn't really make sense with our human biology. Here are her three solutions:

1. *Build a system that reprioritizes doctor/patient relationships so that doctors can spend time with chronic pain patients instead of using prescriptions as a proxy for doctor presence.*

2. *If medicine is our social safety net, we need to give doctors the tools to take care of the problems that really exist instead of biologizing them.*

3. *How about narratives? Can we bring back some of the narratives from 150 years ago? Is it time to do that? How about 'People are resilient'? How about 'The body can heal itself'? How about 'Pain is inevitable… and sometimes useful, if only to remind us what joy looks like'? And most importantly, that 'Doctors are limited in what they can fix once it's broken.'"*[49]

I think that she makes some points worth examining. One that is crucial for Warfighters deals with priorities. Let's ask a question together.

What should we be willing to trade for physical and emotional relief from pain and trauma? The current system says that we should be willing to trade conscious-ness. We should be willing to trade participation in life and love and usefulness. We should be willing to die.

I can tell you right now, that price is too high for any-one to pay.

This is an emergency! We can't wait any longer for that system to change. That's why I'm standing up and saying to everyone who is a Warfighter or who loves a Warfight-er: opt out. Find out the truth for yourself. Make sure that those who fought for us don't get left behind in the teeth of a heartless political and corporate machine.

Bring back the human art of healing.

"The Benzo Battle"

Let me tell you what Johnny's life was like *after* he de-cided to get off the medications that were prescribed for him. Because he did—when my son left Camp LeJeune, he had a heart-to-heart talk with me about his low points and his life and his wants. He did not want to be in a fog of drugs. He wanted to get clear of them.

We had some advantages—I'm aware of that. First of all, Johnny wasn't massively physically disabled. He wasn't paralyzed or missing limbs. Chalk up advantage number one. Number two, I could provide for him. We could give the rating system the middle finger, because I could take care of any of Johnny's living expenses. Num-ber three, I was motivated and naturally prone to question everything.

When I was a young mom, I would take little Johnny to the doctor and sit and listen to everything. I'd watch everything the doctor did with a critical eye. Then I'd take the prescriptions to the pharmacist and have a chat. "What's this one do?" I'd ask, holding up the first one. Maybe it was antibiotics; that was necessary. Okay. "What's this one do?" I'd ask, holding up the second. That one might be a codeine-laced cough syrup. No thanks. I could make a kid some hot lemon-and-honey and give him some OTC pain reliever without using the heavy stuff.

So I had the skill sets to question a VA doctor or just not follow what he said. I could provide the critical eye and healthy skepticism that had been trained out of Johnny during boot camp and four years of service. That was an advantage for sure.

That said, getting off the psychotropics and opioids was not easy for Johnny. Maybe you've never been through that kind of withdrawal or seen anyone go through that kind of withdrawal. It's rough.

First of all, all the things that these drugs are supposed to correct—all the anxiety and physical pain—they attack with full force. You're used to being numb from them; so there's a resentment of feeling like shit all of a sudden that attacks your willpower.

And physically, you suffer. Your blood pressure shoots through the roof. So you're experiencing side effects from that: sweats, headaches, heart pounding, shortness of breath. You feel forty years older than you are. Any activity hurts you.

I ended up in the emergency room time after time with Johnny because his body wasn't dealing with being off the drugs well. He'd be sweating and holding his head, and when they'd measure his blood pressure, you could see the sideways glances or wide-eyed shock from the nurses. He could have had a heart attack or a stroke from coming off that shit.

But he did it. He was young and strong and stubborn, and he had his family with him. So he did it.

What we didn't know is that he couldn't get the effects of the drugs completely out of his system. Here's a fun fact for you in case you didn't know. Benzodiazepines cause non-concussive TBIs. What that means is that these drugs tear away at your brain, just like if you were playing football and getting knocked on your head every single day. Without getting blown up once, you can have the brain damage of a combat vet in serious firefights or an NFL linebacker without a helmet.

True story. I've got some serious research for you later.

That brain damage doesn't just go away because you stop taking the drug. You're not getting any more tears in your brain, and thank Yahweh for that. But the damage is done for good.

You know what a TBI looks like, whether it's from head trauma or not? Here's what. Nausea, vomiting, and other stomach problems. Trouble sleeping. Dizziness. Not being able to concentrate or remember. Headaches. Emotional distress and imbalance. Possible loss of senses like smell or taste.

So you're trying your hardest to stay off the drugs that are tearing your brain apart, literally, and you have to go through that hell on top of it.

For Johnny, it was like a curtain fell between him and the rest of the world. It lifted sometimes, but it was always there, ready to fall back. Here's an example.

I took Johnny and Justin in the summer of 2012 to visit my nephew Chris and his wife Mindy. They are my loves—just genuinely good people that show you what family is meant to be to each other. Chris is a good twelve years older than Johnny, and they didn't grow up together. But when Johnny grew older, he and Chris connected over interests they had in common, like shooting and cars and dogs. They both loved the outdoors.

We did some awesome things together. Chris took the boys to a range to shoot. We all went rafting on the Ocoee River. If you've never rafted before, it can be quiet and peaceful at stretches, but going over the rapids is fast and exciting and dangerous—all the things Johnny had been missing.

You could see when Johnny was having fun that there was a light in his eyes. He would smile. It was like being with the old Johnny again. But he couldn't hold on to the joy. It was like water in a straw basket. You'd mention the rapids later, and he would turn to you with cold eyes and nod without sharing the memory of that joy. He knew he had gone and done something fun, but the fun never lasted for him.

It disappeared behind that curtain.

Johnny got a therapy dog, a Hungarian Vizsla we named Kobe. Kobe would sleep in Johnny's room and follow him everywhere he went. The dog went on vacation with us. He was a good dog, always present, especially when that curtain was down between Johnny in the rest of the world.

Here's another warning sign I should have seen.

In the weeks before Johnny took his life, he put distance between himself and Kobe. He'd put him in Justin's room for the night. He'd complain about him. He stopped showing so much affection for him.

Of course, there was a reason I didn't see this sign. Kobe was really sick and not expected to recover. I thought that maybe putting distance between himself and Kobe was Johnny's way of sparing himself grief ahead of time over Kobe's death. I could understand that. It made sense to me. But that wasn't what was going on.

Johnny was saying goodbye to the whole world. His dog was just really close to the top of the list for him.

So coming home, the part that I saw, was so hard for my son. And as I think about why, I get angry all over again. Angry and then sad.

Coming home for Johnny should have been as hard

as it was for his friend Mike. He would have struggled with finding work, managing relationships, grieving the friends he lost, feeling displaced from military life, and bucking against the lack of progress he would have seen. And he should have been able to rely on counseling and activity and new direction to heal him, like Mike did.

But Johnny came home hurt and then became addicted. So he didn't have the counseling-only option. His body was rebelling against him, and his brain was riddled with rips and tears from the chemicals pumped into him. And compliance was so trained into him that he never questioned the people who got him addicted or kept him addicted. His independence was undermined and restricted consistently.

He was fucked from the moment the first pill went into his gut.

Listen to me, and look for these signs. If your Warfighter is taking benzos and showing signs of a TBI, even though that Warfighter has never had head trauma, get him or her off the meds. Now.

It will be hard work, for you and your Warfighter. But you can deal with it once you know what is going on. Your Warfighter can heal.

I would like to see a difference in the way the VA treats veterans. I would like to see more communication, less automatic prescription, and a transition to natural therapies for a natural human reaction to grief and stress. But I'm not going to rely on the VA alone to make those changes.

That's *our* job.

If you love a Warfighter, it's your job to ask questions. Be the pain in the ass your Warfighter can't be. Do the work of transition.

Support seeking counseling, and give anybody hell who gives your Warfighter a hard time about it. Get your Warfighter in touch with other Warfighters. Recognize the signs of PTS and TBI, and deal with them.

Fight for your Warfighter's independence. Recognize the signs of saying goodbye to the world, and do something. Intervene.

You don't know when all your chances to do something will be over.

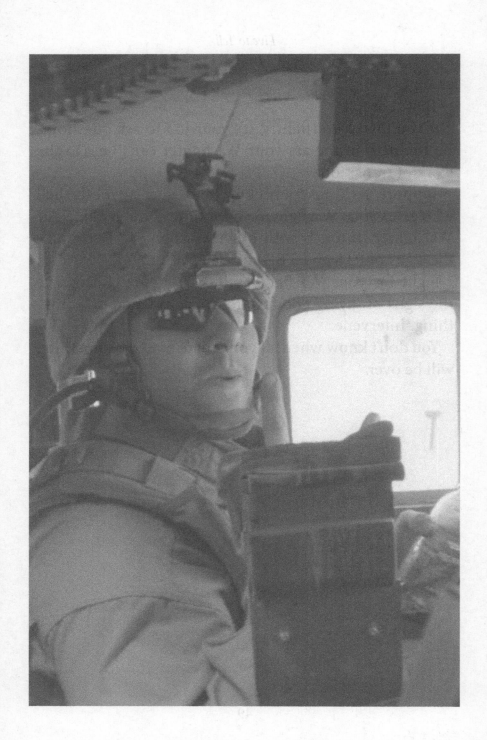

3

Thank You
for Your Service

WHAT really angers me about Johnny's treatment at the VA eight days before his death is that *they all knew better*. It was there in his chart, written in black and white, for any medical professional who cared enough to read it. "Do not give Mr. Lutz Klonopin." They *knew. In fact they have a published report from 2010 on their very own website. It states that you don't treat severe PTSD with benzodiazepines because it causes suicide.*

"Side-Effect: Suicide"

They also knew that Johnny and I had both been through hell together getting him off the opioids. For over two years, I had been supporting Johnny through a physically and emotionally torturous recovery and withdrawal. We had achieved some major gains that cost us both sleep and sweat and tears.

In fact, Johnny had told his psychiatrist at the VA that he had asked me to lock up his guns and pills. And he had. That question showed who my son really was in his heart. He loved life, and he loved his family enough to make sure that he stayed with us. He cared enough about that when he was himself to guard against the possibility that he might not be himself one day. He trusted me to help him in that work.

My son wanted to keep me from the life I'm living now.

So you might be wondering why that particular order about Klonopin was in Johnny's chart. Why did he have a warning against that particular drug? Why was the prohibition stated so clearly?

Johnny had taken Klonopin before.

Klonopin, the retail name of clonazepam, is used to treat two major issues: epilepsy and panic attacks. It works by slowing the neurotransmitters in the brain, mainly a transmitter called GABA (gamma aminobutyric acid). It can cause a host of side effects to almost every system in the body. It can make your heart race, give you the shakes, make you constipated, make you pee too much, and weaken your skeletal muscles, among other things. One of the known side effects is suicide ideation.[50]

But the *main* way it works is by hushing an overactive

brain. In epileptics, that overactive brain causes seizures, and the drug takes away that impulse. In people with panic attacks, the drug takes away the impulse to panic. It takes away control over those impulses. It makes you sleepy and foggy, unable to concentrate.

For some people, especially epileptics I would imagine, this drug may be a lifesaver. I'm not saying it should be banned. If your choices are painful seizures or Klonopin, I'm not going to take it away from you.

But let me ask you: For a young, strong person with no prior history of mental issues, might there be another treatment for panic attacks?

I mean, come on. You look at a Warfighter who's just come back from combat, and you think about that Warfighter as a human person, a normal human person with normal emotions. Like you. Think of yourself. How would you react after seeing people you cared about dying in pain? After seeing innocent bystanders, women and children, made homeless or injured because of the war you're involved in? (The Taliban isn't known for treating its own countrymen gently.)

How would you feel?

You would feel sad. Little things would remind you of people you lost. Ordinary sounds might mimic sounds of trauma. An innocent person speaking Pashto or Arabic in a coffee shop downtown might send your blood pressure through the roof. Crowds might make you think of a crowd that you saw erupt in a red mist and a wall of screams. You would feel angry at what people are capable of doing to other people.

Is numbing those memories and thoughts really the best way to deal with them?

In the confusion and panic of war, maybe. Maybe you do what you need to do to pull yourself together. But when you come home and no one is shooting at you or burying bombs at the side of the road where you walk, shouldn't you have some time and peace to work through what happened to you, what you saw and heard, what you *had* to do?

Shouldn't you be using your brain as an ally instead of sending it to sleep?

Right now, the official VA answer is NO. *If* you're lucky enough to be free of injury and prior exposure to mind-altering drugs, you might get treated like Johnny's friend Mike. *If* you're on top of things enough to ask for counseling with no drugs, you *might* get it. *If* you're part of a VA branch that will actually pause long enough to listen to you, that is. And *if* you have family or friend support enough to help you stick with healing the hard way.

I don't know about you, but that seems like a hell of a lot of *ifs* to me.

When Johnny came home from war, saddened by the violent loss of men he knew personally and scarred by physical injury, the VA doctors looked at him and saw that Johnny was experiencing pain and sadness and sleeplessness. So they medicated him.

Here's a fun fact: if you stop taking a benzodiazepine, your withdrawal symptoms can make your original condition worse. If you started taking them for panic attacks, get ready to stare down the anxiety train. This I know from experience, from watching Johnny. And all of those super enjoyable side effects just shovel coal into that train's engine.

The 2/8 Marines arrived in Camp Lejeune after losing 14 Marines in combat in Afghanistan. The loss hit all of the remaining Marines hard. They gathered in a chapel on base and sat in the cushioned chairs in that dimly lit auditorium looking at the stage. There, portraits of the lost Warfighters stood behind the gun, boots, and helmet displayed in honor of each one.

And after receiving whatever solace each one could take from the prayers and remembrances, they were left to wrestle alone with the dark questions that always follow survivors. *Why him and not me? Why am I alive? How did I make it? What is my life worth that I should still have it?*

Dark questions.

On top of that emotional trauma and his physical pain, Johnny was also left with a broken marriage. Johnny had left for war a married man with a wife waiting at home for him, and soon found out she had been unfaithful and he filed divorce papers. You know young people—especially young Warfighters. In the face of the possibility that you might not come home to do all of the grown-up things later, you rush them ahead of time. And most often, that doesn't work out.

"ALMOST THE LAST DAY"

It didn't in Johnny's case. He moved in with Kevin Ullman, an acquaintance who'd recently reenlisted and been transferred to another unit. But he still hung out with 2/8 guys, playing poker and going out. Kevin was going through a divorce at the same time Johnny was, and that meant that Kevin had an extra room, and he invited Johnny to move in with him.

Not only was Kevin a standup guy, just a good-hearted person who still keeps up with me, but he was also the suicide prevention NCO for the battalion. Johnny needed Kevin around more than anyone knew.

I got on the phone with Kevin to ask some questions about Johnny's mindset in 2010.[51] Back then, I had been trying to give my kid a little space. He was a married adult, and Mama couldn't know every detail. But in Johnny's absence, those details belonged to me. And Kevin was generous in giving me what he could.

Kevin first noticed that something was up with Johnny in 2010, after he moved in. "I knew he was going through some depression and everything. Going through a bad divorce is tough on anybody."

"Did it change him, Kevin? Did he start acting any different?"

Over the long-distance static, Kevin thought before he

56

answered. "At one point I remember he decided to actually stop drinking and go without. He was kind of just being more introverted. That struck me as a little odd, because I'd be like, 'Dang, dude, you want to go out tonight?' And he'd be like, 'No, I'm just going to stay in,' or whatever. At first, you know, we were all going out and doing stuff to keep him busy. He decided to stop drinking, kind of stay in, not really go do anything with anybody."

*Here's another gift of knowledge for you. Don't buy any bullshit excuse for your Warfighter to start staying alone, no matter how good it sounds. To stop drinking, that sounds positive, right? It sounds like a good life change, doesn't it?

Not for a young Marine. Going out to a bar means that you're socializing. You're with people being active, participating in life. You're out of the house, probably showering and changing your clothes regularly. All good things.

When a young Marine like that says that he's going to stop drinking, it could mean something good, I'll admit. He could be going for a full-on Chris Traeger (Rob Lowe's character on *Parks and Recreation)*, obsessed with exercise and organic food and cleanses of one kind or another. It could mean that he's got religion, like Louis Zamperini in *Unbroken*, and he's going to rely on prayer and church services to get him through the bad thoughts.

But it could mean, and it did mean with Johnny, that he's withdrawing. He's isolating. He's burying all of the trauma and anger and disappointment under a numbing fog of prescribed medication, gaming, comfort food, and excess sleep. Maybe random sex, if he's lucky and the drugs have physically left him that option (they don't always, just FYI. If getting some action is important to you, just say no to drugs).

So Kevin would go out to ride bikes or hang with friends or play poker, and Johnny would stay at home doing not much of anything. It was not a healthy choice for him. And Kevin raised the issue one night.

I guess the no-drinking initiative had fallen by the wayside by then, because Kevin and Johnny were having drinks on the front porch of Kevin's house. And Kevin, listening to his Spidey-senses, brought up that depression with Johnny.

"I was just like, 'Look, man, if you end up thinking of hurting yourself or like killing yourself or anything like that, you need to come talk to me, you know?' And we just had a talk about that. And he was like, 'Yeah, no, I'm good, man, it's just—I'm just depressed. I'm in a bad spot.'"

"Because of everything?" I prompted him.

Kevin agreed. "I think it was a combination of deployment and the stress of combat, losing friends, you know, seeing all that. And then also coming home and going through a divorce."

What Kevin heard that night didn't seem like anything out of the ordinary to him. As a suicide prevention NCO, he'd been trained to confront anyone who seemed down and offer that person resources and help. That's what he did with Johnny. Kevin let Johnny know that he wasn't alone, that things would get better, and that there were options for him even if he couldn't see them. Kevin did everything right by the book.

So what happened later that same night was in no way at all his fault.

"We were outside having drinks, and I ended up going to bed," Kevin began. He was matter of fact, like he was delivering a sitrep. But the memory of that night troubled him. "I feel like I was in bed for like five minutes. I must have passed out. And he must have stayed up and had drinks or something, because when he came to my room and asked to use my computer, I was like, 'Yeah,' you know, 'that's fine.' I gave him the password, and I passed back out. I guess his computer was dead. And that's when I woke up to you calling me because he had called you saying he loved you and all this other stuff."

So much happened while Kevin was asleep. From my perspective, far away in Florida, I woke up to Johnny calling me and telling me that he loved me and he wanted to say goodbye and that he now wanted to talk to his brother Justin.

It jolted me awake immediately and sent me into a panic. I could do nothing from where I was. I didn't even know if there was anything left to be done at that point. Johnny hung up, and when I called back, he wouldn't answer his phone.

Kevin did. I remembered him telling me to calm down. I mentioned that memory to him.

"I was like, 'I had a talk with him the other day. He literally was just in my room five minutes ago.' And it had been longer than that, but I just felt like it was five minutes."

And who knows how long it had been? Who knows how long Johnny took to prepare the scene that Kevin would find? Kevin wasn't the only one asleep when Johnny was getting ready to check out. I was, too.

"You got right up when I called," I remembered. "You were really good about that."

Kevin acknowledges my tacit thanks with a small noise. He's keeping his memories in order. "Anyway, I was like, 'I'll get up, I'll get up. Just hold on.' And I went out, and I couldn't find him in the house. And that's when I noted that his pill bottles were scattered from the front porch and into the living room, empty. And that's when I was like, "He's not here. Let me get off the phone; I'm going to try to find him.""

The words no mother wants to hear. They sent me into a numb loop where I couldn't think of what to do next. I was on the outside of what was happening to my son, and my heart was shredding in pieces inside me. I needed sanity and clarity, and I wish I had known that Elohim was as close as my next breath, waiting to offer them to me. Luckily, Kevin was doing all that could be done for

Johnny.

"I called 911 and told them what was going on. I gave them a description of his truck and what he looked like. And then after that, I hopped into my car, and I just drove around looking for him."

"Where did you go?" I asked, picturing myself in that truck beside him, where every atom in my body longed to be.

"I drove around the neighborhood at first. Like, I took a loop around the hood—the neighborhood—and went to the stoplight. Then I just decided to go right. And I just ended up seeing his truck at the gas station around the corner from the house, and I pulled in."

I could see the gas station. I had visited Johnny at Kevin's house once, and I had the look of the neighborhood in my mind's eye. I could see the dark parking lot, the still truck, the motionless driver silhouetted against the convenience store lights.

"He had just, like, drank a bunch of booze and blanked out with his pills. And I just remember opening the door, and I was like, 'What the fuck were you thinking?'"

I could taste the metallic bitterness of that anger and terror and helplessness on my tongue. I felt like that, too, on the last day, in the slowly emptying theater on the last night of Johnny's life. I, too, wanted to scream at Johnny and ask what the fuck he was thinking.

But I know Johnny wasn't the one doing any thinking by that point.

"He was just so out of it. He was like, crying and apologizing and stuff. And I just pulled him out of the truck. By that time, the ambulance showed up. Or the police showed up, because they saw us. And then at that time, they called in the ambulance. And they got a hold of him, got him on the stretcher; they took him off to the hospital."

So matter of fact this man was when he told me that he saved my son's life. It was the next right thing he had to do. He didn't consider himself a hero for finding his friend and getting him help.

"And then I called you and let you know. And I think you were up there, like, the next day."

I remember walking into that hospital room and seeing my son hooked up to an IV, gowned like an invalid. Some of the other guys from 2/8 were there with him. He was still tearful and apologetic when he saw me. He was determined to do better.

Poor guy. He didn't know why he'd had those thoughts, why he'd done what he did. No one explained to him that the Klonopin he was taking to soothe his anxiety was pulling the strings on all the deathward decisions.

Johnny recovered from his suicide attempt and moved back in with Kevin for a few months.

Three months later, Johnny checked himself into Poplar Springs Hospital for treatment of his PTS. He thought that he was helpless against that urge because he was never told that the Klonopin was the cause of his suicidal ideations. With the last bit of his own will that he could muster, he put himself into the hands of professionals. It was the best thing he could have done.

He recovered from that near brush with more suicide ideations on his third day at Poplar. You see, this doctor failed to read Johnny's charts and administered Klonopin again. On the third day, Johnny told his doctor, and that doctor stopped administering it. Then Johnny was good again.

If only the VA had a system in place that notified all treating physicians of drug allergies.

*Here's my next gift of knowledge for you. Every person who's being treated for anything serious needs a medical advocate. Someone who is not the person healing needs to keep track of every prescription, every visit.

Right now, HIPAA laws can restrict your access to medical records due to privacy concerns. So get a medical power of attorney. Get your Warfighter's consent. You can't leave the course of treatment to chance. It's too important, so stay on top of it.

Johnny got better off Klonopin. But it was obvious then that he couldn't put Kevin through the ordeal of having to monitor him and wonder about him. So Johnny moved into the Wounded Warrior Barracks at Camp LeJeune, a place for any Warfighter with mental and or physical injuries.

"After he got out and he moved into the barracks, I popped up to Wounded Warrior Barracks every once in a while and visited him. I saw the room that he was in. From time to time, we'd grab dinner. He wasn't in the Wounded Warrior Barracks, I think, too much longer, because he ended up getting medically retired, medically separated, and then he moved back home to Florida."

Back to Florida—and by now you know the rest of the story there. Now you know why Johnny and I fought so fiercely to wean him from the drugs that were poisoning his mind and his body. Now you know how we both struggled uphill to keep him healthy and free. And how one visit to a doctor who wasn't paying attention and reading the warnings undid two years of hard work.

It makes you wonder again, as I've wondered so many times.

Why this path?

Why these drugs?

Why not try something else?

Look, it's not *just* my son. These drugs are claiming so many lives. Even Vietnam Veterans who have struggled along for years, sometimes self-medicating on alcohol or doing the hard work of counseling, when they start on a regimen of these benzos, they join the suicide statistics, too. These drugs are murdering our veterans at an alarming rate.

"THE ALARMING RATE"

A 2014 story on Military.com noted alarming suicide rates among older veterans, 50 and above.[52] That means veterans born before 1964, veterans who could have served in any military action from 1982 backward. So we're talking about guys who served in Korea, Vietnam, El Salvador, Lebanon, and any number of other operations the guys in DC dreamed up.

The Military.com article suggested several reasons why older veterans may have started dying from suicide. They had probably been using work and family to distract them, and on growing older, they had lost those draws on their attention. They had gone a long time until the VA acknowledged that PTS was real and started treating it. They had been dealing with chronic pain and depression for a long time.

Sure, those are all reasons why someone might fall into despair. But they are not reasons why someone in despair who has survived all those factors for years would only fall victim to suicide after seeking treatment at the VA. The VA prescribes benzodiazepines for anxiety, depression, agoraphobia, stress, and anger. Why doesn't this article make the connection between the sudden introduction of benzos and the sudden occurrence of suicides?

It's more than apparent to me.

Law Enforcement Today reported the terrible, terrible

statistics on suicide among our veterans. They also noted that for each suicide, 135 people are affected, while 48 suffer so much from the impact of the suicide that they require mental or psychological help to heal. Here are those statistics:[53]

1. More than 6,000 veterans have killed themselves each year since 2008, according to the Veterans Administration (VA) data.

2. Veteran suicide rates increased 25.9% between 2005 and 2016.

3. As of August 2018, there were 5,273 U.S. Military deaths since 1999, but there were at least 128,480 veteran suicides since 1999.

4. That's an average of 20 lives lost per day. Only about 6 of them are in the VA system, leaving 14 not associated with VA care.

5. An estimated 150,000 to 200,000 Vietnam veterans have committed suicide since returning home from the war... while 58,315 died in the Vietnam War.

6. The suicide rate was 1.5 times greater for veterans than for adults who never served in the military.[54]
7. Over 1 million veterans suffer from post-traumatic stress disorder and are at risk of suicide.

And those statistics don't even take into consideration the fact that Texas and California, two of our largest states, don't report suicide statistics. Not to mention the fact that suicides occurring in military hospitals are often recorded as secondary combat deaths. The number is much, much higher, but even the reported statistics are absolutely unacceptable.

John Ketwig, member of Veterans for Peace and Vietnam Veterans of America, also notes the lack of clear statistics reporting in many areas, especially in the deaths of Vietnam veterans. Instead of a mental health crisis, Ketwig believes that these deaths arise from a moral health crisis—refusal of society and military alike to acknowledge and mourn the human and civilian costs of war. PTS is not a disorder, but a normal reaction to the horrors of war. He speculates that the fuzzy numbers may arise from a desire not to harm funding for the VA or persuade people not to serve in the military.

Of course, finding and reporting accurate veteran suicide statistics would raise a mass outcry. In the same way, reporting the same, tired, inaccurate numbers has a calming effect. People think that the number is steady—22 a day. There may be a problem, but it's not growing. It's just like cockroach parts in ketchup. There's an acceptable number of cockroach parts that ketchup companies can include and still pass FDA inspection, but no one at Heinz or Hunts is exactly going to advertise that number. People wouldn't buy ketchup anymore.[55]

The suicide epidemic is not limited to the military, either. The Centers for Disease Control and Prevention reported that across the board, over 150 thousand Americans died from drug-related deaths in 2017; over 47 thousand of those deaths were suicides. That's a record. More and more people are dying from suicide, largely because the social structures that used to be present to support them just aren't there anymore.

Danny O'Neel, an Iraq War veteran who survived a suicide attempt, works to replace those social structures. He runs the Independence Fund that he founded to help Warfighters connect with each other and heal the psychic wounds of war through social connection. Danny considers these psychic wounds to be just as harmful as physical wounds, noting that though 9 men in his unit died in country, 15 died by suicide after returning home. One reason veterans default to suicide is the inadequate mental health facilities at local VA hospitals where, Danny notes, some veterans are dying by suicide on the grounds.[56]

In fact, over the past two years, 260 veterans have attempted suicide on the grounds of VA facilities. 20 have died in those attempts. The crisis has gotten so serious that the VA added a third call center to its suicide prevention hotline in 2018. The Trump administration started a task force to study the problem and promised returning veterans mental health help for a year after they leave the service.[57]

What is clear from these stories and statistics is that the VA cannot handle the numbers of returning Warfighters who are suffering in mind, soul, and spirit from the things they have seen and heard and done. Clearly, people who love veterans have to fight for them as they fought for us. Clearly, we have to address invisible wounds—those Ketwig calls moral wounds and O'Neel calls psychic wounds—through helping Warfighters connect with each other. Through that connection, they find healing and hope that they cannot find anywhere else.

"Bad PR"

Despite these terrible, terrible numbers, *nobody* is blaming the drugs or the drug companies. *They blame the veterans.* And that is a severe lack of respect.

There's a whole twisted schtick out there for how people view veterans, and it comes out in three lies.

LIE NUMBER ONE

All veterans are angelic heroes.

We all grew up with the story that all veterans are heroes, right? At least most of us. For a while during Vietnam, if you were a veteran, you were dirt under people's shoes. But the World War II vets got parades, as have some Gulf War and Global War on Terror vets.

Look at pop culture. A lot of hoo-rah military movies have become great hits. You can't even get through Christmas without idolizing a few veterans in *White Christmas* and *It's a Wonderful Life.* Country music? Forget about it. I dare you to name me one major artist without a patriotic music video.

And who *doesn't* love those videos of Warfighters coming home to surprise loved ones? I mean, come on. Just look at the kid at the piano recital lighting up to see her dad, or the old man at the nursing home breaking into tears when he sees his daughter. And don't get me started on the dogs who have been waiting months or years to see little Freddy come back and who practically wet themselves with pure joy when he does.

Those videos and movies and the kind of *Chicken-Soup-for-the-Soul* stories in magazines and online teach us to paint all veterans with the same brush.

But they're *not* the same people.

There are veterans who are great humans and veterans who are not. They're people, the same as other people, only they have a different set of training and experiences. Those experiences and that training bind them together in an extraordinary way, but they don't canonize them.

And the danger of buying into this lie is that superheroes don't need help. They don't need income or medical care or connection to other veterans. They're better than the rest of us, right? Until they can't take it anymore and they join the statistics.

LIE NUMBER TWO

All veterans are helpless invalids.

You know this one. They all come home damaged in some way, and they need to be medicated because they are frail and vulnerable. Poor little cracked eggshells.

Hell, no.

The veterans I know are strong. Even the ones with problems have strength in them. The last thing they need is for people who don't know them and their struggles to talk down to them and treat them like ill children who should be tucked up in bed and kept quiet.

Yes, dealing with dangerous weapons and situations can leave you with trauma that needs to be processed. Veterans who have been in combat need adequate medical care. But what they don't need is people assuming that they can't handle working at their own recovery and taking the choice to be strong out of their hands.

LIE NUMBER THREE

All veterans are dangerous psychopaths.

We started hearing this lie around Vietnam, when the newspapers and television started showing burning villages, naked children, and grimy Warfighters grim with purpose, live and in color. The general American populace looked at that stunning media coverage and thought, "I could never do that! These people in uniform must be

71

savages!"

They forgot their own fathers and grandfathers march-
ing in Veterans Day parades all over America and made
the leap in logic that what they were seeing was somehow
new and different. The media had always shown them
bloodless, sanitized paintings of Redcoats and patriots in
formation or neatly pressed Army green costumes artis-
tically dirtied on the big screen.

So somehow what was happening half a world away in
Vietnam was a different order of war than had ever been
fought before. Only it wasn't.

It was the same damned thing we've been doing since
Cain and Abel. But because of the media and the spirit
of the times, heroes to a lot of people became monsters.

People who adopt this view of veterans want them
medicated, yes. And they also want all of them under
surveillance, known to the police, and marked as the first
suspect at any sign of trouble.

Fuck that.

Here is what I know. All veterans were people before
they took the oath, and no matter what they endure in
uniform or how they come out, they're people after they
come out. We owe them good medical care. But they
don't need worship, pity, or fear.

They need connection.

If you thank them for their service, they'll be polite,
most of them, even though they didn't do anything for
the sake of your thanks. They acted to protect the one on

their left and the one on their right. They did what they were trained to do. A lot of times, your thanks makes them feel awkward. It isolates them, reminding them that there's a wall of difference between them and you. Just letting you know.

And if you ask them what happened to them, for those with visible injury, or what they did in the war—especially if you don't know them personally—just know that you're asking a loaded question.

That visible injury? It may have been gotten in the same attack that killed a bunch of friends. Every time you ask about it, you're making them relive that memory.

That tour of duty? He had to clear an abandoned village, one with a bunch of buried IEDs. People didn't make it. How many details do you want to make him recall right now?

Those memories aren't yours for the asking, just because you're curious. Get to know somebody well before you ask that kind of stuff. Get to know them well anyway.

I have.

It was the next thing I had to find out. What had my son seen that made VA doctors assume he needed medication? What had war been like for Johnny?

What reflections did he see in that dark pool the drugs drew him to enter?

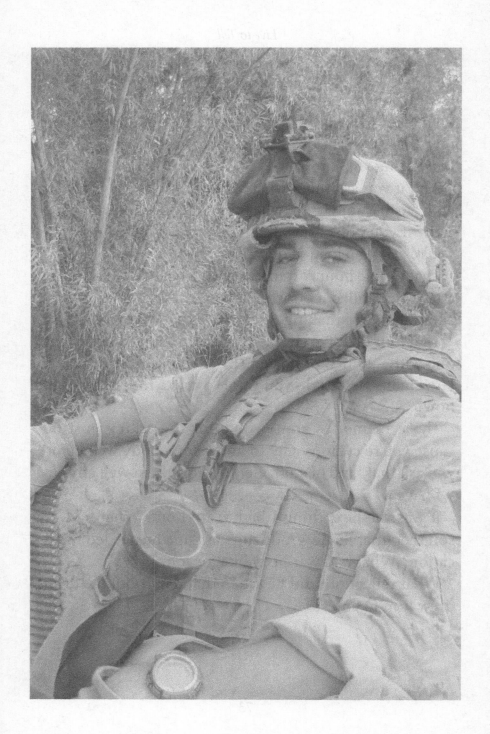

4

LONELY DAYS, LONELY NIGHTS

OVER the years, I kept up with many of the members of 2/8 Marines. One of those guys was Nicholas Rizzo from Boston, known to me and just about everyone else as Rizzo. When he heard what I wanted to know, Rizzo volunteered to go back to that summer and tell me what he could remember.[58]

Probably because of his close relationships with his large family and his tight-knit group of friends from school days, Rizzo had a fairly untroubled transition back home. He didn't make the mistake of getting married before deployment; so when he got home, he lived with his family, went to college, and reconnected with the people who were important to him. After graduating college, Rizzo got a job working for the governor and set his sights on becoming a firefighter—his dream job.

"Rizzo's Gift"

It made my heart glad talking to Rizzo. To see any Warfighter being happy in his life and successful in his career showed me that it could be done. People could go through unimaginable pain, suffer loss, see the worst of humanity in war, and still Live to Tell their stories.

Now it was time for me to hear Rizzo's.

We spoke on the phone, as a flight from Florida to Massachusetts for one conversation wasn't practical. After a few minutes catching up, I told Rizzo we should probably get started.

"Where should we even start?" Rizzo asked.

"Start with when you met Johnny," I said.

"Okay. I met Johnny shortly after I joined 2/8 Echo company in December of 2008. Me and my cohort of new Marines joined the unit on December 19th, 2008, when the vast majority of the battalion was on leave for the holidays. I met Johnny when we returned from holiday break and 'deployed' to 29 Palms for our Combined Arms Exercises, which is a prerequisite for battalions prior to them deploying."

"I remember Johnny talking about those—so you could get used to the desert."

"Yeah, exactly."

76

"And how old were you both back then? I know Johnny was older than you."

"I was 18, and Johnny must've been somewhere in his early 20s."

I calculated backward. Johnny was twenty during the Christmas of 2008, and he'd celebrated his twenty-first birthday in Afghanistan the Summer of 2009.

When Obama took the oath of office in January of 2009, he'd inherited the war in Afghanistan. On the advice of General Stanley McChrystal and Defense Secretary Robert Gates, he'd decided that a massive infusion of 30,000 troops would damage the Taliban so badly that they couldn't come back in any serious way; then Obama could bring the troops home. It was kind of the same idea as Bush's Shock and Awe in Baghdad in 2003.

Only it didn't work that way. We're still in Afghanistan ten years after that decision. And because of that one decision, Rizzo and Johnny found themselves with the rest of 2/8 in Helmand Province.

"And what did you think of Johnny when you met him?"

"My earliest impression of Johnny was someone who could take a room over. He was confident; he was assertive. And he just made everyone laugh. He crossed the line all the time, and a lot of people loved him for it. He definitely pissed a lot of people off, too," Rizzo snickered.

"Yep, that was Johnny. He was a funny guy," I agreed wistfully. An image comes to me of Johnny's face lit up with laughter. It's not a specific image tied to a particular memory I can name, just Johnny being Johnny.

Rizzo added, "He was a Marine's Marine, someone officers and SNCOs probably detested because his cammies weren't always starched and he didn't abide by the day-in and day-out drag of garrison life. The same officers and SNCOs who he pissed off in garrison came to rely on him in combat."

"Why is that, do you think?"

"He was one of those Marines who instilled confidence in those around him, especially some of us younger guys. He was meant to be a combat Marine.

"I'm not going to sit here and say that Johnny was the greatest Marine ever, because he wasn't. Johnny was Johnny. He wasn't—you know how a leader looks at his junior Marines. Because you want your enlisted young infantry Marines to be pit bulls, you know?"

"Oh, I know." Semper Fi!

"So one of these officers might say, like, 'Holy shit, if your cammies aren't pressed, then screw you.' Johnny was not a great Marine. Johnny was a very good Warfighter. Two different things right there. Johnny—he was a calming influence in firefights because that's what he was there for. If I needed someone to talk to a local elder, or with a villager, and again, I was 19 on my first deployment; so I wasn't making these decisions. But I'm not having Janos Lutz talk to a village elder about, you know, what we need to do for their village, because he'd probably just end up

78

telling him to fuck off. And he couldn't even speak any of the Pashtun language. But you know what I'm saying?"

Rizzo has me laughing for real now. Oh, I can just see Johnny in serious negotiations and just turning the whole thing upside down. "I know what you're saying."

"And you know—Johnny and I weren't best friends; he was my senior Marine. But Johnny was friends with everyone, and we had a really good relationship. We became very close on deployment, because me and him had a very similar sense of humor. We laughed a lot and busted balls with everyone."

"I know. I appreciate whatever you can tell me about that summer."

"No problem. So we went to 29 Palms, and then we did some more training when we got back. And then we were deployed to Afghanistan.

"We went to Garmsir (Mian Poshtay) district in Helmand Province. My MOS was Rifleman (0311). Johnny was an Assaultman (0351) in my company and was attached to my platoon and my squad specifically. Him and Jared Paynter, who also tragically took his life not long after Johnny."

"God, what a shame, these boys dying."

"It is. I mean, I don't have a number for you, but in my case, I know my unit's probably lost more guys at home than we did in combat. I think on both my deployments in 2009 and 2011, we probably lost 22 guys. I would take a gander that we've lost more than that by their own hand, you know?"

It hurts me, hearing that. And it makes me mad. It doesn't have to happen, but it keeps happening. That anger refocuses me on telling Johnny's story. I take a deep breath.

"So Rizzo, what was deployment like for you? Can you give me any stories, anything to show what you guys did?"

"We had a very kinetic deployment. I remember when we landed on July 2, 2009, we were expecting immediate and heavy contact by the enemy. But when we landed at approximately 0700 in the fields of Mian Poshtay, it was extremely quiet, and all of the locals departed. We landed in multiple waves via CH53s, which culminated in the largest helicopter assault since Vietnam."

I pictured helicopters landing in green fields, one after another, Marines running for cover—a flood of them.

"We set up a defensive perimeter, and my squad was one of the recon elements that branched out to reconnoiter the surrounding area. Our mission was to seize a bridge that was considered key terrain for the overall mission. Our company had three rifle platoons plus attachments, and each platoon was given a different sector in the defensive perimeter. My platoon (2nd platoon), including Johnny, had the Northern sector, which covered the bridge and the roads intersecting at the bridge code named Route Redskins and Route Cowboys."

I smiled—Redskins and Cowboys. What boys these

were, bringing football onto the battlefield.

"Johnny was at the very northern part of our sector; I was to his southwest no more than ¼ of a football field. Me and a squadmate, Kody Torok, were sent to 1st Platoon's sector to look for a couple of our squad's packs, and it was at this point we started receiving heavy small arms and rocket attacks. I remember hearing the cracks of the rounds smacking over us indicating that the rounds were hitting very close to us and a Rocket Propelled Grenade going over me and Kody's heads, landing about 15 meters behind us and almost killing Sgt Donahue, a Weapons Platoon section leader."

How amazing that Rizzo could talk so calmly and reasonably about bullets and grenades going over his head. I could hear a lot of Johnny in him, when I could get Johnny to talk about the boyhood mischief he got into. But this story was far beyond mischief.

"When there was a lull in the exchange of gunfire, Kody and I grabbed the two missing packs and started to make our way back to our platoon's sector. As we ran alongside the culvert making our way back to the main route, there was a large exchange of gunfire, and rounds were impacting very close to us."

"Good, grief, Rizzo—'Dance, cowboy,' like in the old Western movies."

"I remember this being my first experience with combat and the adrenaline and fear that comes with it. While Kody and I were making our way back to our platoon,

Johnny was on the 240 with Jared Paynter—that was his machine gun, the 240—and I believe they shot something like 10,000 rounds of M240 rounds that day. This was the same day that Seth Sharp was killed in action, by a round hitting him in his neck."

I saw that death, I remember—the death of Sharp. It was in the documentary *Hell and Back Again.* I didn't bring it up because I knew that none of the 2/8 guys liked that movie. They hated that it made our veterans look weak and full of problems. But that death had happened so quickly; it was troubling. You saw how it could have happened to any of them.

"Hey, but just a couple of days later, something funny happened. I think it was July 4th—we had gone into the villages, which was north of where we took our first building. And it was a long day of us searching through compounds. I don't think we got hit that day. And so it wasn't like the first two days in which there was a lot of fighting. After the first two or three days of some heavy, heavy contact, we went through the village, and we were expecting to get hit really hard. We actually didn't. But at the end, or at some point during the day, we're all kind of in a defensive perimeter, and just being like, 'Holy shit, what a crazy last 96 hours!' And all of the sudden, you see Johnny in the back on a fucking donkey, just riding around with the fucking thing. And we all, we all just started laughing our asses off."

I knew the story of the Taliban donkey that appeared

after a firefight and how everyone thought it might have had an IED strapped to it. Everyone had hid until they all realized it was just a lost donkey. What I didn't know is that Johnny rode it. That was EPIC!

"Johnny loved animals."

"He could handle himself around them."

"Oh, I know that. When he was a kid, there was a possum that was stuck in our house. We'd called animal control, called the police. Nobody could get it out. Johnny— like five seconds with a towel, he's got the thing out. And he's holding it up and scaring his dad with it."

"Is that right? Well, here's another one for you, then. I remember we were at OP Empire, an outpost on the western part of our Company's AO and a spot that took a lot of tough fighting to get. There is a video of Johnny somewhere recording a firefight we had at this outpost, and you can hear the artillery in the background that we called in to repel the assault. Anyways, I remember playing chess with Kody, and we could hear something in the walls of the mud compound. Johnny went to investigate, and it ended up being a bat, which started to friggin fly around the room. We were all ducking for cover. It was nuts. I remember looking up and seeing Johnny in his Call of Duty underwear chasing it with a rolled-up magazine. He was swinging at it like he was a professional baseball player the entire time. He finally hit the bat with the rolled-up magazine, and it died on impact. I remember me, him, Kody, and whoever else was in the room laughing about this incident for a long time."

"I can *so* see him doing that!"

"Johnny had such a profound and assertive personality. People like him really make deployment bearable because combat doesn't seem to change them as much. He was so outwardly happy and regular, and I always took it as him being a seasoned vet. During downtime, he was friggin hilarious."

"What else did he do?" I love to hear these stories, the way they bring Johnny back for a moment. This is so him, so vividly him—I can just picture it.

"I don't know if you've heard about this one. Lutz filmed a video of a Huey gun run and 2.75 meter rockets, which is basically when the helicopter goes into attack mode and fires its Gatling gun (something like 3000 rounds per minute). He ended up taking a really good video of one of these runs. He somehow spliced the video of him talking about the gun run on camera as it laid down its rounds upon the enemy, and he said something like: 'Holy shit, look at the size of those rockets! They're huge!' That was the first part of the video. The second was him recording his dick in his hand, and when he talks about the rockets, he spliced in the part of him holding his dick. He kept going around showing everyone this video, and people were under the impression they were watching a gun run attack until Johnny's dick appeared on the camera. Everyone freaked out. It was so goddamn funny. I remember he did it to Sgt Brown, who was a weapons platoon guy turned company intel chief. He did not find it as funny as us, and he bitched out Johnny. Johnny didn't care; he was a Marine's Marine and didn't care about appeasing the senior staff."

"Thanks for that one, Rizzo—what a thing to do!"

"It was really funny."

"But I know it wasn't all downtime. Johnny was in a lot of pain with his back and knee. He got blown up and landed in a ditch. Do you know when he messed them up or what happened to him?"

Rizzo thinks a minute. "I don't recall any specific injuries to Johnny, although if there was anything in relation to TBI, it most likely happened during the firefight that took place on July 17th. I am pretty sure this was the date. Johnny was attached to us during this time, and our squad acted as a quick reaction force (QRF) and reinforced 2nd squad, who was in an extremely fierce firefight to the south of our OP (Combat Outpost Sharp, named after Seth). I remember it being at a Y intersection with 2nd squad to the west of the road in a field strewn out and in defilade (cover), and I was walking point. Sgt Spring, an Assault Section leader, was behind me, as well as my team leader, Andy Bryant, and a couple of Afghan National Army soldiers."

I could see the green fields, with stone walls and tall trees along their bounds, and a grayish white gravel road wide enough for a wagon—or a Humvee. I could see a line of Marines walking one behind the other, looking side to side.

"While we were hugging the road alongside the Main Supply Route (MSR), an IED went off right behind me and instantly killed one of the ANA Sergeants; his name was Mohammed. He was blown over 200 meters into the field. The only reason the IED didn't kill the rest of us that were around the IED is that they were buried too deep, which mitigated the extension of the blast. This blast rocked all of us that were around the detonation. I remember being disoriented by the blast, as well as extremely nervous. Adrenaline kicks in at this point, but I remember vividly one of my squadmates, Cody Hedger, rushing up next to me for cover and yelling: 'HE'S FUCKING VAPORIZED, MAN! HE'S FUCKING VAPORIZED!' This scared me more than anything, because at this point, I didn't know who was hit. A majority of the squad rushed up next to me to take cover on the large piece of defilade that I was on. We found out a couple days later during a company movement south that underneath this defilade were two more 107 Chinese rockets configured into IEDS and as Daisy chains. The initial explosion that killed Mohammed was supposed to trigger the other IEDS, which would surely have taken me, Sgt Spring, and Cpl Bryant out, but the extent of the blast must have severed the connection with the other pieces of munition. We found this out later when one of the Engineers got a ping on his mine detector and found the IEDS."

"What a narrow escape! Seth Sharp must have been looking after you guys."

Rizzo makes a noise of agreement. "If anybody in my squad, including Johnny, had TBI, I would put my money on it being from this specific incident. There were numerous other incidents in which we were close to detonated IEDS, but this one is ingrained in my mind. By the way, this is the IED blast shown in *Hell and Back Again*. Andy Bryant, my team leader, is seen in the video, and Cpl Tran from 2nd squad is the one yelling: 'I told you not to cross here! What the FUCK!'"

"I've seen that one. You guys were in some real danger."

"I remember a firefight in the western part of our AO. We got ambushed, and I remember half our squad being on an elevated platform. The other half, including me and some other Marines, were on the slope walking upward toward the military crest of the hill. When we got ambushed, we naturally took cover as always, but I was in between the enemy fire and the rest of my squad trying to return fire. Definitely some pucker factor during that moment. Rounds were impacting very close, and I had my head down in the dirt trying to get oriented to decide where my next move would be. I remember looking up, and Johnny was yelling at the top of his lungs while Paynter was with him feeding the 240 rounds: 'Rizzo, get the FUCK out of our way!' He was so amped and ready to return fire. I got up and ran as fast as I could to his flank to help return fire as he got the 240 up. Johnny always was calm, collected, and sure where to return fire during firefights. His direction during this moment helped me get into position where I needed to be."

"That's my boy."

"This is what squadmates do for each other," Rizzo explains.

I was suddenly struck with how these men looked out for each other, and how that was all they were doing. They didn't care about any political decisions or any larger goals. They were looking out for each other, for the guy on the left and the guy on the right. The older guys were looking out for the younger guys, just like Johnny looked out for Rizzo. It was a brotherhood, a family.

"You guys were really there for each other. That must mean a lot to you."

Rizzo was quiet. I had spent the afternoon talking to him about some hard memories he would probably rather not dwell on too often. It was time to wrap things up.

"Hey, Rizzo, you've been great letting me in on that summer. Any last stories I should hear?"

"I think I've covered a couple memorable moments so far, and there's definitely many more. One of them is the day Jordan Chrobot was killed in action: September 26th, 2009. My squad went south to try and recon an area south of the Herati Wall. Every time any squad went near the Herati Wall, we got into a firefight. We could tell as we went south we were gonna get into it. You can always tell. The atmospherics of the area change. After a couple of months patrolling your AO every day, you get a 6th sense when you're gonna get hit. The locals disappear. It becomes eerily quiet, and you just feel like you're being watched. Then iComm chatter begins to pick up."

Those details invite you in and paint a picture. I got a flash of somebody in a cheesy movie saying, "It's quiet—too quiet." But I guess every cliché has a nugget of truth at its heart.

"When we got to our vantage point, we got into a defensive perimeter and waited and watched; after an hour or two of nothing really happening, we decided to return to base. I was at the front of the patrol heading back toward base when we got ambushed. The rounds were ripping through the cornfields as the front part of the squad tried to head back toward our defensive positions. I remember jumping into the canal to avoid getting shot. Cornstalks were getting shredded by the incoming fire. When I jumped into the water, the water rushed into my pack, where I was carrying our 119 foxtrot, our radio, and rushed into my magazines. I instantly gained an extra 100 pounds."

Despite the fact that Rizzo was safe in Boston right now, talking to me, my heart was in my throat picturing that scene: the bullets whizzing by, the weight of the water dragging him down.

"I was wading, using all my energy, back toward the defensive perimeter when I heard we had a casualty. My team leader, Andy Bryant, rushed over to me and gave me a hand getting out of the canal, and me and him ran over to Chrobot, Bojo, and Sgt. Mac (the squad leader). Chrobot was hit and was white as a ghost. We knew he was KIA right there. We returned fire. Doc Redman performed a cricothyrotomy to Chrobot under fire (which was one of the bravest things I've ever seen), trying his best to resuscitate Chrobot. I called in the 9-line and got a bird to land for extraction. It took a while, because there was another casualty from an IED in the northern part of our AO. Sgt Gendron was hit by an IED and also needed a medevac. When our medevac landed, we popped smoke, and me, Sgt. Mac, Bojo, and Andy Bryant brought Chrobot to the bird. We were still taking fire at this point. After the bird took off, me, Bryant, Mac, and Bojo repositioned on the southeastern part of our squad's defensive perimeter. Mac gave me the coordinates. I called in a firemission, and he adjusted the rounds. The location where we repositioned was where Kody, Paynter, and Johnny were."

Johnny. I had been waiting for him to appear in this story. And there he was, safe for the moment.

"Johnny was rocking the 240, pouring rounds into the compound and adjacent tree lines where we were taking some of the fire from. At one point, out of frustration at the day's events and losing one of our close friends, me, Kody, Bryant, Bojo, and Mac got on line with Lutz and started shooting as many rounds as we could toward what we thought were the enemy's positions. It wasn't tactical. It wasn't good round conservation, and I doubt we were being accurate. It was an act of frustration and an accumulation of being pissed off. I remember Johnny being in between me and Bryant. Pretty sure he was more visibly pissed off than anyone. Him and Kody were very similar; they always had their emotions on their sleeves. It made them great Warfighters."

A heart on his sleeve. That was my boy. "Thanks for that, Rizzo. Thanks for showing me my boy."

Rizzo deflected my thanks. This was the next right thing he had to do, just as he had done all he had overseas for his brothers. For him, it was nothing that needed thanks—none of it.

Talking to Rizzo had confirmed a few things for me. Warfighters didn't care primarily about politics and larger issues of right and wrong; they cared about their brothers. And as bad as war was, it was a closed community where a Warfighter belonged and knew what to do. Those times saving each other during fighting and making each other laugh during downtime meshed them into a real family. So leaving that community meant that a Warfighter was missing a valuable resource.

Unlike in the past, Warfighters didn't come from the same geographical area and return there; they were geographically isolated on return. Rizzo went home to Boston, Bryant to New York, and my Johnny to Florida— the rest of the 2/8 to different places all over the country. They weren't going to be going around the corner for a beer after work. Community for them would have to be intentional.

And for each of them, it would have to expand to include neighborhood Warfighters from different units and different branches—people who hadn't been shoulder-to-shoulder with them. Warfighters need to connect locally, recognize that they can, and live to tell. Connect-Recognize-Live.

I thought, too, about the impact of those losses—watching Sharp and Chrobot and the rest leave in a medevac chopper. The increasing isolation as more and more men go missing from a unit through wounds or death would be hard to bear. None of them would end deployment with the same unit who left with them. And when they got home, remembering someone no one around you missed would be a lonely feeling. May Elohim give them peace.

After I hung up the phone, I sat on the sofa with my dogs and thought. Rizzo had given me such a gift. And I was one step closer to understanding my son.

"War and Peace"

As a Marine mom, I know that our Warfighters don't do what they do for thanks. Thanks in person are likely to embarrass them; they don't want strangers at Walmart or the post office shaking their hands and making a big deal. After all, our veterans just did what they knew was right. They were just looking out for their buddies on the right and the left.

But a big part of the destructive thoughts that lead people to die by suicide are a sense of hopelessness or pointlessness. When bad medicine starts to work on the brain, it can resort to the lie that the person's life means nothing, that nothing the person has done has meant anything. That is a terrible lie.

For that reason, I'm including a letter from Elham Fanous, a young Afghan pianist.[59] It's important for Warfighters to hear what good has come from their service. And a young man free to lead the life he was meant to have is a wonderful good.[60]

Dear US Veterans of the War in Afghanistan,

Thank you. My simple expression of gratitude seems inadequate, but this seems like the right occasion to try.

I am a 21-year-old student from Afghanistan, getting ready to graduate from CUNY Hunter College with a Bachelor of Music degree. Music is my passion, and playing piano is my life. I will dedicate my career to keeping music alive in places where it is endangered.

When I introduce myself to people in the U.S., often I am the first person they have ever met from Afghanistan. They may have preconceptions about the place and its people that I try to dispel. It is my life's work to put a positive face on my country and to let my art be my voice for a more beautiful world.

93

Afghanistan has a rich and complex musical history, sitting at a cultural crossroads of east and west. In the decades before I was born, my country had a thriving music and film scene. However, all was destroyed in the 1990s civil war, and music was banned completely between 1996 and 2001. This is the world I was born into in 1997. It is a world that would have persisted had the US and its allies not intervened beginning in the fall of 2001, when I was four.

The years since then were difficult and things continue to be challenging. But conditions undeniably improved in my country during the presence of US troops there, to the point that the Afghan Ministry of Education supported the establishment of the Afghanistan National Institute of Music (ANIM), in 2010. ANIM, where I attended school and began my formal music education at age 12, was the first school in Afghanistan in which girls and boys could study music together. At ANIM, students could learn both western classical instruments and Afghan instruments as well as academic subjects. Several of us have gone on to college. Many have become teachers.

The US Founding Father John Adams once wrote, "I must study politics and war, that our sons may have liberty to study mathematics and philosophy, geography, natural history and naval architecture, in order to give their children a right to study painting, poetry, music, architecture, statuary, tapestry and porcelain."

We are those children. You have studied war so that I and my schoolmates could study music. No matter what happens after the drawdown, they can't take that away from us—nor from you.

I can only imagine what American combat veterans witnessed and how they suffered—and continue to suffer—as a result of their service in my country. I have heard about high rates of suicide among young US veterans who served in my country. I wish I could talk to them. I would tell them a generation of young Afghans has grown up in a civil society, which they enabled through their service and courage. I would ask them not to despair that their sacrifice was wasted. I will prove it was not. I will say thank you through my lifetime of music.

Elham Fanous [61]

Elham's letter underscores the point that regardless of the level of military service, all veterans can justly take pride in the undeniable fact that the world is a better place because of the work of the US military. People are free to vote because of them. The terror and torture of secret police ends because of them. Children can grow up free to follow their dreams because of them.

If your loved one ever spouts that utter crap about not being worth anything, show him or her this letter from Elham. And if your Warfighter shows any of the signs of suicidal ideation (I'll outline them for you in the next chapter), then the next section is just for your Warfighter. The Spartan Pledge is literally a lifesaver.

"The Spartan Pledge"

My friend Boone Cutler created the Spartan Pledge with a deeply personal promise between friends. One of Boone's friends had died by suicide, and talking to a third friend about the loss, Boone asked whether that friend had thought about suicide. When the friend revealed that he did almost daily, Boone seized the opportunity to make a mutual pledge that neither one would take his life without calling his buddy first.[62]

That promise grew into the Spartan Pledge. And as the pledge grew and formalized, so did the news of this call to brotherhood to people who take oaths very seriously. Every Warfighter takes an oath when he joins a military service; every Warfighter knows how serious an oath to a fellow Warfighter is. The Spartan pledge states:

I will not take my own life by my own hand until I talk to my battle buddy first. My mission is to find a mission to help my Warfighter family.[63]

Steve Danyluk, a former Marine lieutenant colonel pilot, notes that the Spartan Pledge is not just for those in a dark place. "You don't have to be suicidal to take the pledge. It's finding a mission: Help your buddy. It's reconnecting, re-establishing those relationships that seem to vanish once you leave the military."[64]

One important symbol of the Spartan Pledge is the Spartan sword, forged from the steel exposed on 9/11. Danny Prince, a retired Brooklyn firefighter and Navy veteran, brought the steel scraps to Steve Danyluk, who got those scraps into the hands of Shane Stainton in McKinney, Texas. Stainton forged them into the Spartan sword.[65] Hundreds of veterans have laid hands on the Spartan sword to take the Spartan pledge.

The symbolism of the Spartan sword is hard to overstate. The image of Sparta recalls a culture devoted to war, where not only every warrior but every civilian lived life to support the elite martial class. To say the word Sparta means to remember a place that honored Warfighters and bent every resource to help them in their mission.

A trinity of veterans came together to make it, one with materials, one with vision, and one with skill. And they made it of 9/11 steel. Steel speaks of strength, and that particular steel speaks of a time in our recent national consciousness when our strength was tried and found sufficient. Many veterans signed up for service on that day or inspired by that day. As Boone has said, "Every warfighter in this era is there because of what happened at the World Trade Center and the Pentagon on 9/11."[66]

One quality that makes the pledge so powerful is that it doesn't belong just to one person. It's not a gimmick or a brand. Boone may have written it, but now he says: "I'm just the author, I'm not doing anything with it. It belongs to you now, it belongs to the warfighter community. So the question becomes, what are you going to do with it?"[67]

Veterans are owning that pledge and using it to create their own events and services. The Uniformed Firefighters Association of New York displays the pledge and sword on a page devoted to suicide prevention resources.[68] Spartan Alliance and the Independence Corps makes the Spartan Sword available to veterans for the taking of the pledge.[69]

The Davie PD here locally in my community displays the Spartan Pledge on an easel in their break room. The Nevada Department of Veterans Services held a Spartan Pledge Day in Reno, including food, music, free legal help for veterans, and an opportunity to take the pledge.[70] Warfighters took the pledge at a NASCAR race.[71] Reno's VA held a Spartan Pledge day.[72] Warfighters everywhere are taking the pledge independently at private events and even just among themselves.

What I especially appreciate about the pledge is its targeting of the main problem with pharmaceutical induced suicide: impulse control. Mefloquine interferes with impulse control. Benzos affect impulse control. TBIs affect impulse control. So when the passing impulse to die by suicide arrives in a Warfighter's mind, that Warfighter acts on it without stopping to think.

What the Spartan Pledge does is make the Warfighter stop to think. That's a direct assault against this lack of impulse control. If you as a Warfighter have sworn to talk to a battle buddy before you do anything to harm yourself, then because of your nature as a Warfighter who takes oaths seriously, that oath will come to mind when these thoughts assault you. And in the time it takes you to pick up the phone and call, text, or contact your battle buddy by social media, that impulse has time to pass.

In the moment between the thought and the act, Yahweh has time to work. A new possibility, a ray of hope, a friendly word – our good Father can use any of these to turn aside the final decision for death. The Spartan Pledge is instrumental in fostering these vital moments – these pauses when life is truly on the line.

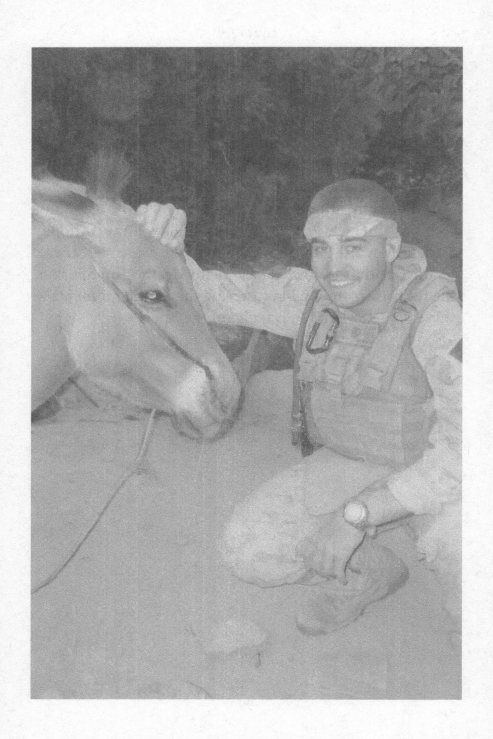

5

IN THE DARK

THE son who came home to me after Afghanistan wasn't the one I'd sent away. Even the son who came home from Iraq showed the beginnings of some changes. I was so busy keeping that son alive that I didn't take the time back then to compare my recollections of who Johnny had been with who he had become.

"WHO ARE YOU?"

Thinking this way made me go back in my mind to my own experience of Johnny after he came home. Of course, I didn't see him for an extended period of time until after his first suicide attempt, when Kevin Ullman called me. So there was a period of time between the time when Nicholas Rizzo saw Johnny emptying his 240 into

101

enemy lines, making outrageous videos, and riding donkeys around for fun, and the time when I saw him in the hospital, when he was sad, remorseful, and emotionally distant.

What had happened during that time? He had suffered grief and anguish over his lost fellow Marines, I know. His marriage had fallen apart, and he had suffered depression. And when he couldn't sleep, he had started taking zombie dope under orders, dope that altered his mind and his emotions.

Obviously, Johnny could handle war. What Rizzo had told me assured me of that. What he couldn't handle was having his nervous system and electrochemical balance fried with prescriptions.

They destroyed him inside long before he died.

I remembered a conversation I had on this same sofa with Danielle, Johnny's high school friend, after Johnny died. We'd been talking about Johnny, and I asked her about the last time she saw him.[73]

"The last time I saw him," she thought aloud. "At that point, I hadn't seen Johnny for some time. I can't remember exactly when it was. I was at a Florida Panthers hockey game with a group of friends, some guys I knew, and afterwards we all decided to go have drinks at this club. It might have been right after Johnny got back from Afghanistan; I know I was over 21."

"I hope you were," I teased her.

"I'm sure I was," she smiled back. "It was really crowded

in there, and I didn't realize that that was probably a red flag for him."

"It must have been. He couldn't stand crowds after he got back," I agreed.

"Anyway, there was a huge bar to the left as you went in with a bull riding place at the back. That's where Johnny was, at the back, kind of in the corner. I saw him, and I couldn't believe it was him."

"Was that because you didn't know that he was home yet or because he had changed so much since high school that you didn't recognize him?"

Danielle frowned in thought. "Maybe a little of both? I'm not sure. I don't think I had heard that he was back yet. And he did look different. Before he left, he was a teenager, and now he had a big beard. He was older looking."

Remembering my son's face, I pressed Danielle for details. "Did he recognize you? Did he know it was you?"

"Yes, definitely," she said slowly, growing serious. "But there wasn't any warmth there. Of course, I didn't realize at first that he was with anyone; I thought he was sitting there alone. That might have made things a little awkward. And me, I'm the type of person who will go up to anybody and say hi. The guys with me didn't know Johnny, but I didn't think anything of saying hi to him."

"I'm glad you did, honey. What was he like? How did he seem?"

"I went up to him and said, 'Hi! How are you?' and he

gave me a short answer like, 'Good, fine.' He was emotionally just not there. The old Johnny would have gotten up and given me a hug, and he didn't."

"I know. I noticed that change, too. He used to be so friendly, and so warm around his friends. What you're describing—that was a complete personality shift."

Danielle nodded in agreement with me. Clearly, her last memory of Johnny wasn't her favorite. "He was not welcoming, not okay. I said something like, 'I can't believe you didn't call me and let me know you were home! We should hang out!' because that's what Johnny would do. I was shocked that he didn't reach out. He was the type of person who would always reach out to his friends."

"He was, Danielle; he was," I mourned. My son's love and warmth had been stolen from him while he was still walking around. It was wrong. It was sad for both of us.

Her eyes filling with tears, Danielle had leaned her head against me. "It was just cold and weird. So I left. I had no idea that's the last time I was going to see him. I wish I had known. I wish I had known what was going on with him."

Those words of Danielle's echoed in my mind after my talk with Rizzo. What a difference! From a prankster and jokester, Johnny had turned in a very short year into a robot.

Those thoughts agitated me, stealing the warmth I'd felt on the phone call with Rizzo and filling me with anger. So I got up and put Stella on a leash. I needed to move, to work out some of this rage and frustration so that I could come back to this line of thought later.

I walked my neighborhood in the blazing heat until some of the heat went out of me. I started noticing things—palm trees, flowers, floats bobbing in swimming pools, people's cars and which ones needed a wash. I slowed down and let Stella sniff grass and take care of business.

Then a car passed me, driving slow. Inside were a group of teenage girls on their way somewhere. They had their phones out, of course, and they were shrieking over something on one of them. I heard only a snatch of conversation. One girl said, "So gross! Why would he take that?"

Her words brought up another conversation I had with Mike, Johnny's high school JROTC friend who'd joined the Navy.[74] He'd been talking to me and some other people after the funeral, all sharing random memories and wondering who noticed what and when. It's natural at a time like that, I think, to compare notes and speculate on what we all could have done differently.

Someone had shared a comment Johnny had made, and in response Mike had said, "Oh yeah, the most jarring thing he said came after Afghanistan. He was back home. Me, our friend Andy Penta, my then girlfriend, her friend, and Rafael Pellerano went to Quarterdeck, a restaurant where a friend worked. I was still in the Navy, and Andy was still in the Marines. So the three of us were talking about military stuff at one end of the table."

Heads nodded. Some guys from 2/8 were in on this conversation, and they knew how conversation just naturally turned to battles and military life with Warfighters off duty. You can't just turn your brain off, especially when you're around other Warfighters.

"We got to talking about the nasty shit John and Andy saw during their deployments," Mike remembered, "and you could tell Andy didn't really want to talk about it. John started showing us pictures of dead combatants he and his unit had come across."

Mike looked up at me apologetically, hesitantly, asking silent permission to share this next part. I nodded at him.

"He showed us really messed up pictures of disfigured, burned and decapitated bodies, and I could see that Andy didn't really care about it. He looked away from the photos and started talking to the other people at the table. I was more fascinated with John's reaction to the pictures. He didn't act like he was showing us dead bodies. Instead, it seemed like he was showing us pictures of puppies or something like that; it was weird."

It was weird, yes. But it was also understandable. I could understand the impulse. If you saw something unbelievable, even something unbelievably gross and disturbing, you might want some photo proof that those images weren't just something twisted up inside your head. You'd want some proof that it was real.

Looking at some of the guys he didn't know well, Mike

explained, "This was totally not like him in high school. He was a little competitive; he was a guy. But he wasn't obsessed with fighting then."

"You guys were in JROTC back then, right?" someone asked.

Mike nodded. "There's a strange dynamic in JROTC programs, maybe in ROTC, too; I don't know. Some of the people know they're going to college ROTC. They're really serious about the program and really competitive about leadership and doing well in there. But some of the people in there know they'll enlist. For them, they say that all the training is fake, that this isn't the real military. So they don't take the program that seriously. That was Johnny. He wasn't a dirtbag about it, but he wasn't ambitious. He did what was beneficial to him and left the rest."

"So showing these pictures, he wasn't trying to one-up you guys? To show that he was more of a badass?"

"No, absolutely not," Mike said. "He used to tell me I was badass with my job, and I was like, 'You're the badass.' No, it wasn't like he was trying to prove anything or gleeful or obsessed or anything disturbing like that. He just didn't make the connection that these weren't things you showed other people. It didn't register with him."

Those words had jarred me—it didn't register. I thought of how many times over the last months of his life things just hadn't registered with Johnny. Joy. Anger. Interest in things he had loved. They had all just washed by him like debris in a flood. The capacity to salvage anything meaningful was extinguished. The memory was painful. I wish now that I had been able back then to reach out to Elohim for strength.

I brought myself back to the story Mike was still telling. "Andy told him, 'I'm on leave. I don't want to see this crap at home.' And he switched seats. After that night, I talked with Raff and Courtney, and we all commented on how weird that was. I realized that night that something was different; something had changed about him."

"What did you see that changed, Mike? Over time, what was different?" I asked.

Smiling sadly, Mike confessed, "I thought he was a clown when I met him. The first time I ever got internal suspension was with John. In fact, a lot of first times happened with John. We were a bunch of jokers, and we were invincible...nothing could hurt or stop us."

God, that hurt—thinking of those young, swaggering boys ducking each other in my pool or walking down the sidewalk outside school. They were invincible back then. I wished I could have frozen time for them.

"That initial impression of John didn't change for a while, not until he got back from Iraq," Mike said. "Johnny grew up, but so did all of us. It would be weird if we all stayed the same as we were in high school. I remember that we were all still in the military, and our friend Andy was home. We decided to go hang out at Raff's house like old times, and John looked at me and said, 'This looks like a pretty irresponsible group of people' and got up and left."

The circle around me broke up laughing. I could tell that each and every one of them could absolutely hear those words in Johnny's voice. I know I could. He'd probably said something exactly like that to many of them.

Mike wiped away some tears of laughter. "Obviously, this was enough for me to go to Raff and tell him what happened. Johnny came back with his gun and his silencer and started to put it together. John and Andy went to a corner and started to talk about the ballistics of the gun, and they straight up discharged a weapon in the backyard of my best friend's house!"

The laughter broke out again, all of us remembering Johnny, picturing his mischievous grin when he came back into the house.

"All of our girl friends were pretty alarmed, but we just shrugged our shoulders and thought, 'That's John,'" Mike sighed as he finished that story.

"So different from the Johnny that came home after Afghanistan and showed you those pictures," I noted.

"Yeah," Mike agreed, shaking his head. "He was still himself then, after Iraq. He was still pulling pranks, finding some humor in being with us. That wasn't like the shell-shocked guy that pulled out those pictures."

"But that humor sounds a little different from high school," I mused aloud. "A little sharper, a little more dangerous."

"True," Mike admitted, "but maybe that was just the

growing up part. Maybe that's the sense of humor we would have gotten to know if we'd had more time with him the way he was."

The way he was—if he'd never started taking that damned zombie dope. Sitting there at Johnny's funeral, I had been so mad that I wanted to scream and throw chairs around. But I controlled myself. I balled my fists and just fumed.

The remembrance of that intense anger brought me back to myself. It was time to head home. The walk had burned the frustration and fury out of me by now, and Stella needed some water. The day was intensely hot.

I made it home, took care of Stella, told the other dogs hello, and got a drink of water for myself. I had done a lot of remembering today, and the memories had worn me out. But I didn't have time to rest. The phone rang, calling me back to daily life. Super Stone needed me to make a decision; I made it and hung up.

Holding that phone in my hand, I remembered standing just there and hearing Johnny's voice on the other end of the phone. He had been deployed to Iraq. I hadn't heard from him in a while; so a phone call was something to celebrate, something to make me jump up and down and laugh with happiness and relief.

If you love a Warfighter, you know the pure joy that floods you when you hear that voice and know that everything is okay, at least right now.

But when I got over the giddiness of the fact that my

kid was okay and talking to me, I asked how he was doing. When he answered, he sounded guarded. He sounded like he was choosing his words carefully.

"I'm okay," he started. "There was a car bomb the other
day and we were the first to arrive on the scene. There
were body parts scattered."

And then my boy whispered into the phone. It was
barely a breath, so soft that whoever was listening beside him might not have heard it. He probably meant for
whoever was beside him not to hear it. But I knew what
he said, and it sent chills down my spine.

He'd whispered, "Be careful what you wish for."

Oh, God. He had wanted to be a Marine so badly. And
once he made it and learned all the fighting techniques
and the Warfighter mindset, he had wanted into the fight.
He wanted to make a difference. He wanted to be the one
to fight the terrorists that attacked America on our soil,
to do so well that he'd work himself out of a job. He wanted it to be real, all of it.

And now it was.

"Be careful what you wish for." As I stood in that sunny
kitchen with my phone in my hand and my son dead for
six years, I could still hear his words as clearly as if he'd
just whispered them across the ocean.

He'd been so brave. All the letters Johnny had sent home
were basically cheerful. He never complained about the
135-degree temperature, the dust, the food, or any part of

his mission as a Marine. Instead, he kidded his brother. He sent his love to me. He wrote messages for the dogs. He wished he could be swimming in our pool, eating an ice cream.

Just that one crack in the wall, that one whispered message, showed me how real his wishes had become. Just that once, I heard in his voice that what he was seeing was not okay, that the broken bodies and spilled blood touched him and shocked him and grieved him terribly. I never heard him say anything like that again, and I sensed when I saw him again that the last thing he would want would be for his mother to bring up that whisper, that moment of revelation, when he was home again and surrounded by familiar people and normal things.

I couldn't wish that Johnny had never become a Marine. A grown-up Johnny who hadn't followed his dreams and his great big courageous open heart wouldn't have been my Johnny. But I found myself thinking over some of the conversations I'd had since I'd gone looking for Johnny's story and wishing that some things could have been different for him.

One big thing out of the way—I wish he could have stayed single. And that's not just a snarky jab against his former wife. It's a realization that people like Mike and Rizzo, people who deployed as single men, didn't have the stress of caring for a wife back home while they were fighting. They could come home and work on themselves. They could figure out their anger issues and their grief and pain alone without considering the needs of another person, or as in Johnny's case, the painful end of a marriage.

So that's something I wish could have been different for Johnny when he came home. Also, thinking of high school friends like Danielle and Mike and Courtney and Raff and so many others, I wish that Johnny had reconnected with them more. I wish he had relied on them more and confided in them more.

But maybe he just needed other Warfighters around. Maybe he couldn't open the Iraq can of worms around people who hadn't seen inside that can before. If Johnny could just have spent some directed, purposeful time around other Warfighters when he came home from Iraq, maybe he would have had a better time coming home from Afghanistan. Maybe he would have found a better way to deal with the carnage and horror he was seeing than snapping a picture to prove it was real.

I wished he could have been living with me instead of Kevin, as completely awesome as Kevin is. I pictured Johnny in the local *Lutz Buddy Up* during the program, talking to Warfighters from every branch who were all coming home to Davie, Florida, and who all could understand to some degree what Johnny was feeling and thinking because every one of them, too, had gotten what they wished for.

This I knew: what happened to Johnny in Iraq changed him. It shocked him to his core. It made him a little more desperate, a little more reckless. It led him to some bad life choices. It put some distance between us for a while that I wish I could go back in time and erase.

So here is a little gift of knowledge for you. Notice those changes in personality. Don't ignore them; they're not all just natural growing pains. Encourage your Warfighter to talk and connect locally to other people in the military community before there's a problem.

You don't want to wait until the sleeplessness is so bad that drugs are on the table as a treatment option. You don't want to wait until the isolation and escapist numbing behavior takes over. You don't want to wait until the one you love is staring down that dark pool and trying to stay away from the edge. You want to do something way, way, earlier than that.

You want to do something when you know for sure that the person you love is no longer the person who left home. When you see that first crack in the wall. When you feel that first lurch in your heart. When you hear that first whisper from the other side of the ocean.

"HIPAA HELL"

One roadblock for me personally when I got Johnny home and went to work helping him get well was HIPAA. I was in charge of making sure Johnny stayed alive. I was in charge of taking him to the emergency room with bad reactions to VA meds lingering in his system.

But when a relative drove Johnny to the VA right before his death, HIPAA made sure that I knew nothing about that visit. Not about the Klonopin that would drive him to die by suicide. Not about the desperation of his mental state. Nothing.

All that was private.

Congress passed the Health Insurance Portability and Accountability Act in 1996, when the Internet was brand new. It consisted of five parts, or titles, each addressing a specific issue: Title I, health insurance coverage for workers moving jobs or losing a job; Title II, standards for electronic transfer of information; Title III, guidelines for medical savings accounts; Title IV, guidelines for group health plans; and Title V, guidelines for company-owned health insurance plans.[75]

The act itself is good and well-intentioned. No one wants some sneaky sneak to lift social security numbers and insurance information and sell it on the black market. In fact, the act outlines some pretty hefty penalties for violations. "State attorneys general can issue fines up to a maximum of $25,000 per violation category, per calendar year. OCR [the Department of Health and Human Services Office of Civil Rights] can issue fines of up to $1.5 million per violation category, per year. Multi-million-dollar fines can be—and have been—issued."[76]

A Breach Notification Rule requires providers to notify all patients that they are following a breach—another added expense. And criminal charges may be levied after an investigation by the OCR.[77] So violating HIPAA could break a medical practice, send health professionals to jail, or bankrupt the doctors. Those are very good reasons for medical professionals to take privacy seriously.

HIPAA protects several different kinds of information, all falling under the definition of Personal Health Information (PHI). "PHI includes a patient's name, address, birth date and Social Security number; an individual's physical or mental health condition; any care provided to an individual; or information concerning the payment for the care provided to the individual that identifies the patient, or information for which there is a reasonable basis to believe could be used to identify the patient."[78]

There is an exception for patients to grant access to a friend or family member to know the information in a medical file. You should know that HIPAA right and act on it to help your Warfighter get the proper care.[79] My only problem with this rule is one of common sense. What if the health problem is suicide ideation? And what if one symptom of suicide ideation is hiding the chemically-induced intention until it is too late?

My son had a good plan in place with one VA doctor. He told the doctor that he had given me his medications and weapons for safekeeping. Johnny was off the benzos and making strides. Then things went sideways for him, and when he showed up at the VA less than ten days before his death, he contradicted everything he had said previously. After that appointment, no one kept me in the loop.

If it was in Johnny's chart that he had designated me to hold his drugs and guns and that he was trying to stay off meds, why didn't anyone there let me know before replacing the drugs he had previously surrendered?

This is what I would like to see. I would like to see civilian caregivers and physicians working together on a veteran's team. Once someone is trusted and looped in, that person should be notified of psychological or medication changes. We shouldn't be playing games with what a trusted ally is and isn't allowed to know about veteran care, especially when we are dealing with suicide ideation as a side effect of a prescribed medication.

We need a little common sense here.

Another thing you need to understand is how the nature of HIPAA works within the culture of the military, especially the Marines. They're Devil Dawgs. They don't know what pain is. They don't need comfort. They learn that in boot camp.

You have to understand that in order to be a Marine, you go through a hell of a lot. Now basic training is hard in any service. And some elite groups in different branches have even tougher training, like the Green Berets or the SEALs. They are some dangerous, no-joke folks who go through unimaginable pain shaping themselves into the fierce Warfighters they are.

Having watched from afar as my boy went through Parris Island and came out the other side, I can tell you that training a Marine—any Marine—is an iron forge that melts and molds the raw metal of human flesh into the mirror-surface cavalry sword of a Marine.

Drill instructors control the way you eat, the way you sleep, the way you walk and move and talk. The training almost breaks you down to a state of infancy and then grows you up into a different kind of being in a few short weeks. And this training doesn't exist just for bragging rights. No.

The Marines need to know that when they send a unit to do a job, that job is going to get done the way they expect. They need to predict with absolute accuracy the result an order is going to produce. They have that predictability down to a science. By the time any Marine sets a foot on a field of battle, the questions are drummed out of them. Yes, sir is second nature. It has to be. You stop to question, and your brother dies. They *all* know this.

So, two things are going on here. One—by the time the Marine Corps has shaped a man into a Marine, they have invested a lot of time and training into that Marine. They are going to expect that Marine to be a Marine as long as he is capable.

If a Marine gets injured on the field, he's evaluated. If he's still able to serve, he gets whatever he needs to keep going. In a moment of crisis, Marines patch each other into shape to get the mission done. You're in pain? Take some painkillers. Your head's not right? Take some uppers and *OoRah* the hell out of here.

This didn't happen with Johnny; he didn't return addicted. After he came home, he couldn't sleep, and the VA prescribed zombie dope for him then. But that same training made sure that he wouldn't question anything he was given and instructed to take.

I had originally assumed that Johnny returned from war injured and stressed out and grieving, and the VA doctors discussed what had happened to him and came up with a treatment plan with him. That's a wrong assumption on so many levels.

Two—in addition to military culture that accepts pain as necessary, you need to consider the compliance instilled by training. By the time the Marine Corps has shaped a man into a Marine, that Marine is unquestioningly obedient to his superior officers. Now, put him in a bar with a few buddies, and you'll swear your Marine has never heard the word *compliance* in his life. But put him in a doctor's office with a medical man who outranks him, and you've never before seen anyone swallow a pill faster.

Nobody's discussing anything with you if you're hurt in the field. Nobody discusses anything when you get back. You're an object in this treatment plan, not a subject. And the same thing continues stateside. You're already on A, B, and C? Fine. Keep on. And add X, Y, and Z, too.

To assume that a Marine is going to question a VA doctor who outranks him is to operate in a fantasy land. That Marine is so trained to accept orders that he literally *can't* do anything else. He doesn't ask what potential side effects are. He doesn't ask whether there are other alternatives available. He doesn't ask whether the drug is really necessary. He says *Yes, sir* and fills the prescription.

And he takes it. Did you know that the VA will test a Warfighter's blood for the presence of the drug he's prescribed? They will. They're making sure our veterans aren't dealing painkillers for the extra cash. Nice view of our veterans, huh?

And if they don't find evidence of that drug in the Warfighter's blood, he can lose his rating. The rating system, for those of you that don't know, measures a Warfighter's percentage of disability and provides him living expenses according to that percentage. If you're not taking your drugs, the reasoning goes, then you must not need them, and if you don't need them, then you're all better. So, you don't need any provision.

Bullshit.

"TBIs, OR THE NFL WITH GUNS"

Besides not being able to say no to a prescription, Warfighters also battle physical difficulty keeping up with prescriptions. Why? It's all wrapped up in head trauma— Traumatic Brain Injuries. And remember: taking Mefloquine causes a vestibular TBI that's not caused by a blow to the head. Chances are that any Warfighter deployed on foreign soil is suffering one of those, whether he knows it or not.

The work of Dr. Bennet Omalu caused a sensation in 2015, when Will Smith starred in the movie *Concussion* based on Omalu's autopsies of football players with repeated head trauma. These football players, beginning with Pittsburgh Steeler Mike Webster, experienced mood changes, problems with judgement and impulse control, and other psychological symptoms before early death. Omalu traced the symptoms to microscopic tears in the brain over time.[80]

Like football players, Warfighters get knocked down, brush themselves off, and keep going. Over a single deployment, they may encounter multiple IED blasts, falls during firefights, or other head traumas. And remember, the Mefloquine they are required to take overseas causes microscopic damage to the brain, creating non-concussive TBIs.

The American Association of Neurological Surgeons says that about 1.7 million cases of TBI occur each year, and that 5.3 million people currently have a disability from head trauma. Around 235 thousand people go to the hospital to be treated for brain injuries every year, and the costs of their injuries total between $48-56 billion annually.[81]

During a TBI, some force strikes the head. Inside the skull, the brain sloshes in its cerebrospinal fluid from side to side. That motion may tear tissue inside the brain, or it may cause a bleed inside the brain or into the fluid, all depending on how severe the injury was. Immediately after the injury, the brain will start to swell in an effort to keep the brain from moving anymore. If the swelling is too severe, a patient may need surgery to relieve pressure on the brain.[82]

After the injury heals, patients experience a range of symptoms, again depending on the severity and location of the injury. Some patients eventually develop degenerative neurological conditions like Alzheimer's, Parkinson's, or dementia. Though some have to learn basic living skills like talking, walking, dressing, and feeding themselves all over again, others will suffer milder but more long-lasting symptoms.[83] The CDC categorizes those milder symptoms into four areas: thinking (memory and reasoning), sensation (sight and balance), language (expression and understanding), and emotion (personality changes and social inappropriateness).[84]

The Mayo Clinic recognizes a whole host of symptoms. Physical ones include dizziness, altered senses of taste or smell, vision problems, headaches, tinnitus, hearing loss, headaches, seizures, problems swallowing, and facial paralysis. Intellectual symptoms include problems processing information, making decisions, problem solving, and multitasking, in addition to problems with memory, judgment, learning, reasoning, organizing, planning, concentrating, and completing tasks. Communication problems include difficulty speaking, writing, organizing ideas, using muscles to form words, understanding words, understanding nonverbal cues, staying on topic, modulating proper tone and pitch when speaking, and trouble following and participating in conversations. Behavioral symptoms include risky behavior, difficulty with self-control, problems in social situations, emotional changes like depression and anxiety, lack of empathy, sleep problems, difficulty recognizing objects, skin tingling or itching, and verbal or physical outbursts.[85]

A study done at Walter Reed and reported in the *New England Journal of Medicine* reports that "soldiers with mild traumatic brain injury reported significantly higher rates of physical and mental health problems than did soldiers with other injuries. Injuries associated with loss of consciousness carried a much greater risk of health problems than did injuries associated with altered mental status,"[86] such as seeing stars, feeling dizzy, or being unable to recall the events before or immediately after the injury.

And the *Journal of Head Trauma Rehabilitation* agrees, stating that "traumatic brain injury can result in long term or lifelong physical, cognitive, behavioral, and emotional consequences. Even mild TBI, including concussion, can cause long-term cognitive problems that affect a person's ability to perform daily activities and to return to work. As a result of these consequences, TBI is one of the most disabling injuries. Although similar to that for several other types of injuries, the percentage (15.7%) of injury-related productivity loss attributed to TBI is 14 times that associated with spinal cord injury, another important disabling condition."[87]

With all of the symptoms of TBI scientifically proven and medically known, it baffles the mind to realize that VA doctors expect veterans to keep up with complicated dosage schedules for up to thirty medications. Nothing is wrong with me, and I'd have a hard time with that! How in the world is a veteran with a TBI supposed to deal with it? For the sake of practicality if nothing else, veterans should have a civilian counterpart who has access to HIPAA-protected medical information and who can ask questions of medical staff and manage a treatment plan.

And to help soften some of the symptoms, you can follow some of the recommendations of the American Occupational Therapy Association at home. To compensate for memory trouble, you can encourage the use of planners, checklists, cueing systems, and technology. Use labels everywhere, on cupboards and drawers, to reduce frustration. Rely on schedules and routines, and discuss emotional changes and low frustration tolerance openly.[88]

But for the love of God, don't just organize all the VA pills in a handy container and think that the problem is solved. Remember that suicide ideation is a side effect of both benzos and TBIs. Involve your Warfighter and all the people close to him or her in recognizing the signs of suicide ideation and bringing any that you see out into the open.

"Signs of Suicide Ideation"

When you are looking for clues that someone you love is thinking about suicide, you may feel frustrated; after all, you're not a mind reader. Add to that the fact that our service members are predominantly male and that men are less likely to talk openly about feelings, especially dark ones. So, you should pay attention to what you can see and hear: behaviors and statements.

Let's start with behavior. We can divide behavior into actions and nonverbal cues like gestures and posture. How does someone who is contemplating suicide behave?

That person will cut contact with people and/or pets, write a will or a note, act recklessly, give away special possessions, increase alcohol or drug use, search for information on suicide on the Internet or through TV programs or books, and gather materials to use for the suicide.[89] Those are big, obvious gestures. When you see those, time is running out fast.

But maybe you're not finding the notes or the Internet history. What nonverbal cues can you see? Think about irritability, anger, anxiety, shame, and depression. How do you act when you feel those things?

The cues to those feelings can look like lashing out verbally or physically, knocking things over and slamming doors. They can look like refusing invitations, disengaging from social media, not bathing or showering or changing clothes, or changing eating patterns. They can look like pain relief behaviors, like shopping, napping, eating, substance abuse, sexual promiscuity, or over-indulgence in video games or TV or Internet browsing. They can look like mood swings, being happy and outgoing and then sad and withdrawn with no perceptible reason for the change.

You can also look for signs of agitation like wringing hands, putting clothes on and off over and over, or pacing. Depression can look like not finding joy in things that used to bring it, like exercise, food, sex, or socializing. And besides behaviors, pay attention to what statements you do hear. People at risk may wish they had never been born. They may tell people goodbye.[90]

You may hear big statements like, "I wish the world would end." But you may hear other statements, too, that you shouldn't ignore. The person may talk about feeling hopeless, being in pain, feeling trapped, or not having a reason to live. The person may talk about being a burden. You may hear a lot of revenge statements.[91] They may seem paranoid. They may talk about life for other people when they're gone.[92]

One huge warning sign that suicide is imminent is a sudden relief or happiness after a period of depression. I'm not talking about a baby step in the right direction; I'm talking about obvious giddiness. The person could say something like, "Everything's okay now," or "You don't need to worry about me anymore."[93]

If you see some of the big risk factors like plain statements or preparations, you need to act immediately. Here is what you do. You stay with the person; don't leave him or her alone. Ask for help from family and friends to keep the person company if you need to. Stay calm, and help the person stay calm, too. Ask the person to give you weapons, drugs, rope, or whatever materials have been gathered to cause death. Call 911 or get the person to the emergency room. If the person is in treatment, also call the psychiatrist or therapist.[94]

However, maybe you're not at that stage. Maybe you're just seeing some behaviors and picking up on some words and gestures that worry you. Ask them if they are thinking about suicide and if they have a plan. If they have a plan, then this is something we need to take very seriously. This is where we remove access to what is included in their plan. Find an anchor for them that will keep them focused on something they love, like their child, dog, or that special person in their life. If you have more time, you can do some proactive things to help the person. Make sure that the person has access to good medical and psychological care and that he or she has a good relationship with the providers. Do all you can to deepen the person's relationships to family and friends. Promote cultural and religious beliefs and practices that are life-affirming and discouraging of suicide. And restrict access to materials for death like drugs and weapons.[95]

One thing that you need to keep in mind is that preserving your Warfighter's life is not your full-time job. Warfighters must own and participate actively in preserving and caring for their own lives. Yes, there are things you can do and things you should notice. But the most important thing is your perspective. Preventing suicide is not something you are doing to your Warfighter; it is something you are doing with him or her.

With that in mind, the National Suicide Prevention Lifeline suggests some veteran-specific approaches that veterans own proactively. One of the first is to involve family and friends in your thoughts and feelings. That can sound hokey and selfish to a veteran. You can let your veteran know that it's not: that you care and want to hear what's going on.

Further, the veteran needs to talk to other veterans about what's going on. That unique community knows what the veteran has experienced. Because of that common history, they can talk more effectively and specifically about service-related grief and anger.

And finally, the veteran should make a safety plan with certain steps that he or she can follow. The plan needs to be something automatic that the veteran will know and can do. And friends and family should know it and be involved in helping. A safety plan may look like calling a buddy, locking up materials, going to a designated location, or calling 911.[96]

Keep your eyes open. Do what you can do. And rely on the inner strength of your Warfighter to act ahead of time to preserve life.

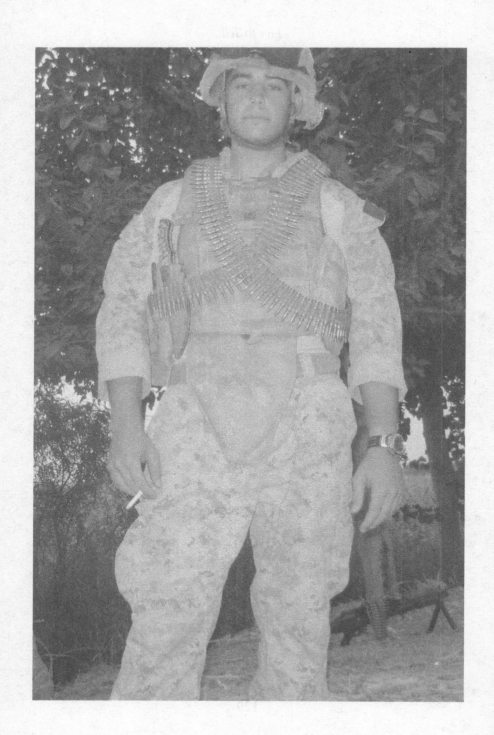

6

Broken Tools

BEING a Marine Mom is something that I am very proud of. And being the mother of an 0351 Assaultman makes me stand just a bit taller. You see, my son was born to be a Warrior, and he got that warrior spirit from me. He is bone of my bones and flesh of my flesh. I say to all the moms out there who birthed children that stand up and fight for their country: Stand tall and be proud! Our children are the warriors of this great country, and we birthed them. So, take pride in that fact, and know that it all started with you.

"PsyOp"

After I made the decision that I was going to fight for those that fought for us, I realized that I needed to educate myself on what was really going on in the Warfighter community. I had heard about a squirrely PsyOp'er named Boone Cutler who had his own radio show called *The Tipping Point*. He was a published author and a Warfighter. I started listening to his show, and as soon as I heard the intro, I knew I had struck gold. His intro starts, "Much to my surprise, not everyone everywhere shares my opinion. I am Boone Cutler, and what you hear is what you get. So, if you have a complaint, send it to me, Boone Cutler. The time is now; the place is here. Why am I here? Cause I'm going to tell you the Warfighter perspective." Bam—it happened just like that. I found a Warfighter who is an influencer and who understands the race against the clock in saving our military family. After I began listening to him every Saturday, I learned that my son wasn't the only one to die of pharmaceutical induced suicide. Many have died of pharmaceutical induced suicide, but many have overcome.

On the 1-year anniversary of John's passing, I held an event to raise awareness for PTS and a memorial motorcycle ride. I reached out to Boone and told him what I was doing, and he invited me on his show. When we did the show, he learned about Johnny, and it was then that Boone and I became connected. You see, Boone also almost lost his life the same way.

Boone parachuted into a dangerous place and spent 2005 and 2006 working psychological operations for the Army. His job was playing real-world military and mental chess with people on the street. He was in a sense a puppet master of the most dangerous people, pulling their strings. After coming home wounded, Boone went to Walter Reed, where he stayed for two years. After making it through and getting back on his feet, he knew his mission was to help his Warfighter family, and the radio show was where he started.

Over the years, when I had a new idea about an initiative I wanted to create, I would call Boone and run it by him. As is only natural when you have mutual respect for each other and your mission is aligned, you become close. And being that we are both military, him with his time in service and me with my Marine son, the rest was history. I became part of Boone's immediate family, and I love him like a son. I don't say this as if he is replacing Johnny, as no one could ever replace him. I say this as a Marine Mom who is proud of another Warfighter. The love I have for Boone and our community is a beautiful gift that I have been given. The ability to give and receive love within my military family is powerful. It is also a gift from my good, good heavenly Father.

Anything major that I heard or that I wondered about, I would call Boone because I wanted his perspective. And after I won the battle of Mama Lutz vs. The United States Government for wrongful death of my beloved son, Boone was the first person I called.

He couldn't believe his ears. He said, "Do you realize what this means for our community?"

I said, "Yes!"

Then he shared with me, "I was your son." He told me then that the pills almost got him at Walter Reed.

It was that very moment that my #IwasLutz initiative was born. When Boone stated to me that he was just like my son but survived, I said, "I want to collect stories. I want to hear who else died of pharmaceutical induced suicide, and more importantly, who survived." I wanted to share these success stories with the world, and I wanted to know how they did it. That is how and why #IwasLutz was born.

I spoke with Boone the first time in 2013, and finally I met him in person in 2019.[97] It was time for me to wrap my arms around him, his wife Malisa, and his beautiful family that of course included his three furbabies: Ajax, Sushy, and Gorgo. Just another thing we have in common is that we are both dog lovers.

We sat down on a spring day at his kitchen table. It was early in the season and still cold out. I could see some lingering snow drifts from his back patio against the hills, where a pale white sun was beginning to descend.

I enjoyed dinner and good conversation with his beautiful family. After dinner, the family cleared off and left Boone, Malisa, and me at the table to talk over water, tea, and slices of homemade banana bread. This was a surreal moment for me.

I couldn't believe I had Boone and Malisa all to myself, and I was relishing it. I loved them, and I knew they loved me. We all knew that we had each other's backs."

Have you ever experienced being able to speak and share, knowing that the people you are with are just like you in the most important ways? That whatever you say and whatever response you get, you know without a doubt that it is coming from a place of love? I don't say this lightly: When your mission is truly aligned with no hidden agenda and you are not living by your ego but by a shared ethos, nothing but good can come from that place.

Boone leaned back in his chair and took a drink before smiling wryly across the table at me and asking, "How you really doing, Mama Lutz?"

I couldn't help but laugh before we both grew serious. Boone could see something behind the smile. I replied, "This is a tough time of year for me, Boone, with birthdays, Mother's Day, and Memorial Day coming. I'll be okay; just waiting for it to pass."

Boone and Malisa both got up and sat on both sides of me, letting me know that I'm not alone and that they were going to get me through the funky funk.

Now our conversation turned to a critical moment of my son's care. Johnny was prescribed two contraindicated drugs on that fateful day of his last VA visit. Morphine and Klonopin should never, ever have been prescribed together, yet they were. "Why is this happening in an age with so much technology available at our fingertips?" I vented.

Boone said, "You know that military secrecy is kinda my thing, right?"

I nodded. "Sure, and coming from you, I'm sure you're about to make an important point."

"So, I'm going to ask you to look at things from the military point of view, right? You've got to understand: the military exists to do a job. All its resources, all its mind power—it all goes to that job. Now, they keep pretty good records. But as far as sharing those records—no. What you get from the military is on a need-to-know basis, and they figure that they're the ones handling the treatment. So, they're the only ones who need to know what's going on. You start opening up military records to civilians on request, and where does it stop? And the paperwork? That's another nightmare waiting to happen."

We sat in silence for a moment. Boone could sense that his words were not enough of an explanation for me.

"You've seen pictures from Afghanistan, right?" Boone then asked me. "You've seen the women in burkas?"

I nodded.

"They say it's for a good reason," Boone shrugged. "It goes beyond modesty for them. The woman belongs to her family—even the sight of her. Only her husband and female relatives ever see her unveiled. And they say it's for her own good. From their point of view, they're protecting her. She's hidden. She's not tempting anybody. It keeps her safe."

"Pretty uncomfortable, too," I add, only half-joking.

Thank God I was born in the USA!

"My point is, you have this whole cultural tradition that's trying to do something good. It's good to want to protect women, keep them away from guys that might want to hurt them, take advantage. I think even you'd agree that's a good goal."

"Okay."

"It's just the way they're going about is very extreme. That's the same thing with HIPAA. It's a medical burka. The government is trying to do something good, protecting privacy. You don't want your social security number out on the dark web, right? You don't want anyone using the details of your identity and your medical history to stick you with a huge bill after some criminal gets surgery or deals pills on your dime. The government's just going about privacy in an extreme and totalitarian way. They're not considering the unintended side effects."

I looked out the window and pondered the thought of the side effect not being intended. The sun was descending toward the hills, turning the whole valley rose-gold. It was a heavenly sight, and I wanted to sear it into my memory.

I realize that Johnny was trained to follow orders, and in combat, following orders saved his life dozens of times. There's a reason questions and pushback get drilled out of you in boot camp, no matter which branch you join. In a serious situation, you can't have some yahoo debating what comes next. No. You get your ass over the wall or down the road or into the building, and you don't stop to think why. People who don't fall in line get killed more often.

I know that this is part of the problem when they come home. I express this frustration to Boone, how something else good, this training, isn't working on the outside. More unintended side effects.

"It's not their job to make it work here. That's *our* job." Boone inserted.

Those weren't just words, coming from Boone. He had given up a good, secure job to advocate for Warfighters on the radio and to lobby lawmakers on veteran issues. He'd suffered personally in many ways as a result of making that decision. But he had decided that acting for his Warfighter family was the best use of his life, and he wasn't going to back down.

As I sat at Boone's table, I thought about the ways that coming home is hard for a Warfighter. Separation from a close-knit group of colleagues. Finding a new job. Healing from wounds—body and soul. Adjusting to the civilian pace of life. Thanks largely to the zombie dope, Johnny didn't make that transition. Boone, after some rough patches, did.

"I've been thinking about the transition phase, Boone. You already know that this time of year especially, I think about what went wrong and what we could do better."

"I think about that, too," Boone said. "Almost every day, I've got a guy calling me up to help him through that re-adjustment."

"What I'm hearing and from what I remember, the civilian world is kind of like an alien planet when a Warfighter first gets home. They've been on planet military for years, where they're used to the way things work, and then they get marooned on Planet Civilian. There's a different gravity. Everything seems slow and complicated to them. They can't just get things done; they have to do them the way civilians say. It's like trying to thread a needle while wearing a spacesuit. It makes things hard."

Boone nodded. "It is slow—you got that right. After running for your life on a regular basis? Yeah, filling out forms online for a job feels like death."

"I remember how Johnny used to get frustrated at simple things sometimes. He didn't want to plan a trip ahead of time. He didn't want to get into the details, the budget, the stops. He wanted to decide on two or three things and then just get into the damn car."

"I hear you," Boone nodded. "'Get into the Damn Car'— good title for a manual on transition."

"But there isn't one—that's just it. When Johnny came home, nobody told me, 'By the way, your son has experienced X, Y, and Z, and it's changed him in these specific ways. So, you're going to have to relate to him in a whole different way. And also, look out for these drug side effects. And also, look out for these signs of intending suicide. It would be nice to be told."

"Who's going to tell you? Every other military family is

just coping the best they know how. A few organizations are helping raise money for the wounded and for suicide awareness, but proactively dealing with the transition period? Forget it. That's why they need us."

I sighed in frustration. "The world, most of them—they have this expectation that Warfighters will just jump back into the flow. Hurry up and fit in now, get better now, get over it now. But they can't. It's unrealistic. The government should want to spread some public awareness about that."

Boone shook his head. "Look, the military is there to fight wars. They make a significant investment in each Warfighter, with training and housing and clothing and pay and the rest of it. So, when that Warfighter's job is done, the military just wants to cut its losses. You ever hear about DRMO?"

"Sounds familiar, but I can't place it right now."

"It stands for the Defense Reutilization and Marketing Office. You have a chair in use fifteen years that isn't great but isn't broken, and the DRMO sells it and makes room for a new chair. Jackets, computers, weapons, anything that isn't really useful anymore goes to DRMO and ends up in the Army-Navy surplus stores. The Armed Forces routinely dispose of items that cost more to repair than replace; this happens with Warfighters, too. It's not some evil plot; it's just efficiency."

"It's hard to wrap my head around that point of view. These are human beings."

"I know that, Mama Lutz. They are human beings who matter. That's why you and I do everything we do."

"So, the military sees a guy retiring, gives him his walking papers, and waves goodbye to him. It's not enough. There ought to be more done."

"Yeah, but the government isn't going to do it. We're in a situation where we can bang our heads against the wall all day every day trying to get congresspeople to change things, or we can just do the work ourselves. We can work to change some laws, sure. But in the meantime, I'd rather do the work myself. I've got a big mic, and I'm not afraid to use it."

The last sentence came out like some dramatic line from an action-hero movie, and it made me laugh. Then I frowned. "You know one thing that really bugs me?"

"What?"

"The people in non-profits who are spreading the word about veteran suicide—they're all toeing this line with the 22 a day statistic."

"I know that's bullshit. They don't even count Texas and California."

"Two of the largest states! I know!"

"And the guys who die in VA hospitals on that zombie dope get counted as secondary combat deaths, not as suicides. That skews the number, too."

"I know," I told him, my frustration mounting. "But you know what bothers me the most? All these people saying that the number is 22 a day almost creates this expectation with the VA and the public and other veterans. Like, we already know that we're going to lose this number; so let's all just accept it and move on."

"That's sick."

"It is sick. It's not acceptable to lose one a day, and people are being desensitized to the whole tragedy of it."

"And I hate to say it this way, but speaking of the DRMO, just from a numbers perspective, the suicide epidemic is an acceptable loss for the government. Allowing it to continue makes smart fiscal sense. Cuts down on VA expenses, and lower government spending makes some voters happy."

"I read recently that there's a date in the future when the VA is going to shut down all benefits for World War II veterans. I guess they figure that if you've made it this far, you can make it the rest of the way on your own."

"That's what happens when people become numbers before anything else. They get treated like numbers."

"Transitioning Home"

Each year, around 200 thousand service members go through some kind of transition assistance program. The first real transition programs appeared after World War II, as part of the GI Bill. The first counseling as opposed to pure benefits packaging began in 1991, when troops demobilized from the Cold War and the Gulf War. This kind of separation counseling became mandatory in

2011. The VA acknowledges the importance of a successful transition in helping to prevent veteran suicide.[98]

Every branch of the military offers some kind of transition assistance, which is conducted through the Department of Defense. Different branches call the training
different things, and each puts its own stamp on the material.

The Army Soldier for Life Transition Assistance Program emphasizes civilian success as an Army duty to reflect well on the service.[99] The Air Force is cutting transition program requirements for reservists and giving
airmen the option to complete some training on You-
Tube.[100] The Navy calls its program *Transition GPS (Goals,
Plans, Success).*[101] The Marines offer a program called the
Marine for Life Cycle which includes a *Personal Readiness
Seminar.*[102]

The process starts with filling out a DD-2648, a Counseling Checklist. This form gets a service member an
appointment with a counselor to talk about goals and
strategies to reach them.[103] Also, a service member gets a
DD-2586 or VMET, which verifies the relevant military
experience and training.[104]

The core transition material for all separating service
members springs from the same format. For five days,
Warfighters complete workshops in adjustment to the civilian world, financial planning, understanding VA benefits, and pursuing a career or education. The DoD offers
additional two-day modules in starting a business, going

to college, or finding a career that capitalizes on military skills.[105]

The transition program focuses on practicalities like writing resumes, interviewing, networking, and preparing a profile that includes experiences and preferences.[106] However, these programs take place at military bases, which are not the places where service members will be entering civilian society.[107] After attending the mandatory program, only 15% of service members attend the specialized modules at all, and only 2% start the whole program more than 90 days before separating.

So, the Department of Defense is making some changes to its TAPs, mostly to make sure that service members begin the transition process earlier. Beginning in October 2019, every service member in any branch will meet with a counselor to design a more personalized transition in one of three tiers of services, from most help offered to least. The transition process will begin no later than a year before the end of service.[108] The Capstone, which ensures that all the material is complete, will have to occur no less than 90 days before separation.[109] The VA is also beginning a female-specific transition program to focus on dealing with women's issues.[110]

However, these transition programs cannot see real success until they occur in the veteran's hometown, connecting him or her to the actual people who can hire or enroll them or provide medical benefits locally. They will also not see true success until the VA benefits portion emphasizes alternative therapies for stress, depression, anxiety, and insomnia instead of defaulting to zombie dope.

People who think they want to die aren't looking for a job.

I brought up transitions with Boone at his kitchen table. I had my own ideas of what worked and what didn't, but I wanted Boone's opinion. So, I asked him.

"If you could do the transition process differently, Boone, what's one thing that you would do?"

Boone thought only a moment before he answered. "One thing that would be so easy it's almost stupid not to do it is to hold back on the DD-214 and the transition programs until they get home."

"Oh, Boone, this is a great and a very doable plan. They could do their transition program at their local VA Vet Center and get to know about the place. How I wish I had known about the Vet Center when John was alive! The Vet Centers provide the best counseling. They offer one on one, group, marriage, grief, and MST counseling. They have yoga, tai chi, and many other natural healing modalities. Here they can start their process of healing without the dangerous psychotropic drugs that the VA likes to hand out like candy. These drugs are not dealing with the real issues; they are only damaging their bodies, suppressing their emotions, and causing suicide ideations and suicide. They are actually hindering our veterans' readjustment to civilian life."

"I know it," Boone agreed.

"The families need to get more involved in the healing process then, and if medications are prescribed it should only be temporarily. The families should know what medications their Warfighter is taking and what all the side effects are."

Boone replied, "At home, they'd be transitioning with other vets from different branches who live near them. They could have people from the local college or university explain how the GI Bill works with that specific location and giving them contacts for the actual people they'd have to talk to."

"You've got it. Right now, they go through transition removed from the real life they're going to have to live back home. I think that should change."

"That's a great idea, Boone."

"Mama Lutz, we need to make that happen sooner than later. So, what's one thing you would change?"

"So many things. Prescribed pharmaceuticals should be a last resort. I know not being able to sleep, anxiety, and hypervigilance are three huge problems for most of our returning Warfighters. I say that they should try cannabis first for all of these symptoms while effective treatments are being adopted to purge the trauma from their bodies—modalities such as Elohim's breathing, yoga, and tai chi, just to name a few. Every veteran that has a TBI should immediately receive 40 dives in a Hyperbaric Oxygen Tank, which is proven to heal their brains. So, let's give it to them sooner rather than later. Boone, you and I both know that the pharmaceutical industry is not for our benefit. It's all about money. I believe that our bodies are made to heal themselves if you give them proper rest and nutrition, and if you put everything in there that we need. With the new science of epigenetics, I know that their mindset is the most important. Epigenetics says your environment, your perception, and the way you think, whether it be positive or negative, affects us biologically. Also, these Warfighters should come back and just be together for like, six months. You know? And just stay together and talk together."

"So that they can work things out together."

"Yeah, just let them be together, because it's going to be different for everybody when their stuff comes up. Some people's stuff will come up right away. For others, it'll be months. For some, it could be even longer than that down the road. But you know, talk about the feelings that they're going to have. You know—get real about it. Medicine is not the answer. PTS is not a medical condition. It's a human condition."

"That's right. If you take away the wounded—and hell yes, get those brothers and sisters every medical intervention in the book—then nobody's sick here. People are sad or angry about what they saw go down. Let them work it out."

"Like people, not like lab rats."

"You got it, Mama Lutz. No more lab rats on our watch."

Boone looked at me seriously across the table. "Mama Lutz, you and I are going to make it happen. We are going to change the world for our family."

I replied, "That's right, Boone. Together we will!"

"Continuing Mission"

After I left Boone and went back home to Florida, I kept thinking about our conversation. Once veterans transition home, they've got to learn how to be at home. They need something to work towards. They need a mission.

Veterans have a saying based on that phonetic alphabet they all use on the radio. It goes "Charlie Mike," and it means *Continue Mission.*[111] A veteran hearing Charlie Mike from another veteran will recall a whole host of associations—memories of specific times when going forward with a mission seemed difficult or impossible, yet they did it.

Veterans have huge reserves of stamina, skill, and determination. Charlie Mike reminds veterans of who they are and what they can do.

Former Navy SEAL Alden Mills calls Charlie Mike "an attitude of action." He calls for people to find a mission and stick to it with the perseverance of a SEAL.[112] Veteran community service organizations The Mission Continues[113] and Continue Mission[114] both use the phrase in their names. The security headhunter organization Silent Professionals uses the phrase as a call to spare no effort finding a good job and acting in accordance with military values while doing that job.[115]

The phrase Continue Mission implies that the mission is one that the Warfighter already knows and has been doing, and it also contains the understanding that this mission continues in the civilian world, which is an entirely different sphere from the military. So, what is it that Warfighters are supposed to continue doing in the civilian world?

Look at the Oath of Enlistment for all enlisted members of the military: "I, _____, do solemnly swear (or affirm) that I will support and defend the Constitution of the United States against all enemies, foreign and domestic; that I will bear true faith and allegiance to the same; and that I will obey the orders of the President of the United States and the orders of the officers appointed over me, according to regulations and the Uniform Code of Military Justice. So help me God."[116]

Even though veterans are no longer obeying any direct orders from officers, they still can support and defend the Constitution. The Constitution lays out a lot of guidelines for what the United States should look like. When was the last time you or the veteran you love read it? You both could find a lot of great ideas for life after the service in there. And the United States has a lot of enemies, foreign and domestic, that could use a good dose of opposition. You only have to look at the daily news to see what those enemies have been up to.

Find something that rings your bell and go to it. You can take a shelter dog for a walk and throw a ball for it. You can plant trees or pick up trash by a trail or the coast. You can spend time with inner city kids and show them how they can overcome a hard situation. You can provide for the homeless, protect victims of domestic violence, or listen to the elderly. America is full of people who need a veteran's attention to Charlie Mike.

The point is to be involved and to be relevant. Think of the society that World War II vets built after they got home, the safe and prosperous years of the fifties and sixties. General John Wainwright, a leader during World War II, wrote a letter to soldiers leaving the Army after that war which details what he saw the continuing mission to be.

HEADQUARTERS FOURTH ARMY
FORT SAM HOUSTON, TEXAS

To: All Personnel Being
Discharged From The Army of The United States.

You are being discharged from the Army today—from your Army. It is your Army because your skill, patriotism, labor, courage and devotion have been some of the factors which make it great. You have been a member of the finest military team in history. You have accomplished miracles in battle and supply. Your country is proud of you and you have every right to be proud of yourselves.

You have seen, in the lands where you worked and fought and where many of your comrades died, what happens when the people of a nation lose interest in their government. You have seen what happens when they follow false leaders. You have seen what happens when a nation accepts hate and intolerance.

We are all determined that what happened in Europe and in Asia must not happen to our country. Back in civilian life, you will find that your generation will be called upon to guide our country's destiny. Opportunity for leadership is yours. The responsibility is yours. The nation which depended on your courage and stamina to protect it from its enemies now expects you as individuals to claim your right to leadership, a right which you earned honorably and which is well deserved.

Start being a leader as soon as you put on your civilian clothes.

If you see intolerance and hate, speak out against them. Make your individual voices heard, not for selfish things, but for honor and decency among men, for the rights of all people.

Remember, too, that No American can afford to be disinterested in any part of his government, whether it is county, city, state or nation.

Choose your leaders wisely—that is the way to keep ours the country for which you fought. Make sure that those leaders are determined to maintain peace throughout the world. You know what war is. You know that we must not have another. As individuals you can prevent it if you give to the task which lies ahead the same spirit which you displayed in uniform.

Accept that trust and the challenge which it carries. I know that

*the people of America are counting on you. I know that you will
not let them down.*

*Goodbye to each and every one of you and to each and every
one of you, good luck!*

J. M. WAINWRIGHT
General, U. S. Army Commanding[117]

Wainwright encouraged returning soldiers to lead
when they returned. It's an idea that still holds water.
People who have not served look up to veterans. A veteran can speak up against injustice and be heard when a
civilian's voice won't be heard. A veteran stepping up to
the challenge of public office automatically has a right
to speak on issues concerning the military and foreign
policy. No sheltered college boy in government will ever
be trusted on those issues in the same way as a veteran
will be.

Having these advantages in skill, trust, and personal
gravity makes a veteran a valuable and desirable asset to
the community at large. People desperately need the experienced input, practical wisdom, and mental strength
of veterans, even if they don't know it. Serving as a teach-
er, policeman, first responder, or charity volunteer can
spread the word of veteran value and help to change
some negative stereotypes.[118]

Think of the deeply divided and racially charged atmo-
sphere in politics right now. Military veterans in every

branch have the advantage of having served in a racially balanced and equal organization. That experience alone is invaluable to work anywhere.[119] Maybe if more veterans took charge of government, they could get everyone to calm the hell down and use their common sense again.

Also, what is important for Warfighters affected by the plague of pharmaceutical induced suicide is that Continue Mission is a way forward. It's a way out of the dark thoughts that poisonous drugs put in your head. It's a strong rope of connection to life and to purpose that can fight against the terrible lies that zombie dope will tell you.

The Mayo Clinic lists 6 benefits of volunteering. It can: 1) lessen the risk of depression, 2) give you a sense of purpose, 3) keep you active, 4) reduce your stress, 5) help you live longer, and 6) keep you connected to other people.[120] Harvard Medical School also says that volunteering can lower your blood pressure.[121] And volunteering can be a way to let you have fun or try out a new career without making a commitment to expensive education or training.[122]

If you want to be purely selfish about Charlie Mike, you can be. It's good for you. Though volunteering is more beneficial when the motives are purely to benefit others, going into it with your eyes on a prize for you still wins you many of the same physical health and mental peace benefits.[123]

We all know that civilian society can be frustrating for

a Warfighter returning from military life. Civilian society can seem slow and complicated and frustrating for a person who is used to lying in wait for enemy combatants, running away from enemy fire, and expecting hidden explosives every time he steps outside his door.

That's why we see our Warfighters turn into adrenaline junkies. They want to drive fast cars, chase gorgeous girls, shoot loud guns, watch horror and action flicks, and play violent video games. Those are all sources of adrenaline. They relieve the frustration of not facing death daily.

And as impatient as Warfighters are with civilians, it seems that civilians are just as impatient with Warfighters. I see little civilian willingness to do the hard work of understanding the veteran perspective and adjust to veteran needs. There seems to be an attitude of expecting the Warfighter to hurry up. Hurry up and get over your PTS. Hurry up and fit in with all of us. Hurry up and stop needing medical and psychiatric services.

Hurry up and get over it.

But that's the wrong attitude entirely.

"A Way Forward"

I have a vision for how Warfighters can thrive at home. I know that they are incredibly valuable people that America needs. We can't afford to lose one more Warfighter to this horrible epidemic of veteran suicide. So here I'm going to share with you a practical way of life for anyone affected by PTS.

MY SOLUTION
FOR THOSE LIVING WITH PTS

1. Connect Locally with Veterans. Peer-to-peer meeting is a great way to express yourself and not have to worry about what might come out of your pie hole. Civilians do not understand what they have not experienced.

2. Find a Local Accountability Partner. Look, we all need someone who we respect and trust to run ideas and thoughts by. When we have "stinkin thinkin," we need to hear someone say, "No, that is not the way it is," or "Where the heck did you get that idea from?" Also, your AP should be someone who has overcome similar experiences and is healthy. You can use a color-code system to communicate with your AP and others how you are currently doing:

1. Green-Everything is ok.
2. Yellow-I'm triggered, anxious and/or angry.
3. Red-I'm disconnecting from life.

3. Write Down What Your Triggers Are (i.e., crowds, loud noises, etc.). This is really important. Sometimes, we don't realize why we are mad, short-fused, and reactive. We can slip into Code Yellow subconsciously; we react to things without even realizing it. So, when you and your family learn your triggers, it's a win-win! The time it takes to manage triggers will vary by each person. Taking action on your own behalf leads to the road of recovery, and eventually you will laugh in the face of those triggers!

4. Calendarize Your Trigger Dates. These would be dates that you experienced trauma or loss. Having your family and friends know your trigger dates is a sure way of you not being allowed to isolate for extended periods of time. We all know that the negative side of isolation can lead you down the rabbit hole into the funky funk, which can then lead to the disconnection of life and / or Code Red. Code Red is when you are isolating and disconnecting from the people and things that you enjoy in life. Maybe you have always loved fishing, but suddenly now you hate it. You get where I'm going with this. This is very important for your friends and family to be aware of.

5. Tell Your Family and Friends These Dates and Have Them Set Up Reminders for Themselves 6 Weeks Ahead of the Specific Date. This literally saved my life. I have a friend who has all my dates in her phone. She pays a bit more attention to me and makes sure that I don't isolate for extended periods of time. One day, I had planned to check out. My friend showed up at my house with the cops because she knew something was awry. Of course, I denied it all. I said she was being over reactive. Then someone said it was my son's birthday, and I just broke. I didn't consciously realize this, but subconsciously my body felt it all. What I have learned thus far is that knowing why I feel the way I do at specific times of the year helps me to know what I need to do. This is a good time to hang with your peers. Some days, I just wait for it to pass when I can't overcome it. Other days, I'll focus on an attitude of gratitude. An attitude of gratitude goes a long way.

6. *Reduce or Stop Alcohol Consumption Until You Have Learned to Manage Your PTS.* What goes into your body affects your mind, and you need your mind to be sharp so that you can be in charge of dealing with your PTS. If you stay in an alcohol fog, you're giving your power away.

7. *Voices in Your Head.* If you become aware that you are hearing voices that are directing or compelling you to do things that you know are wrong, contact your accountability partner immediately.

8. *Detoxify Your Mind and Body from All the Toxins and Prescriptions You Have Been Given or Taken Since Your Time in Service.* Also, you need to stop all negative self-talk. Make healthier food, and drink more purified water. Daily infrared sauna, exercise, yoga, Elohim's breathwork, positive affirmations, practicing mindfulness, acupuncture, prayer, and journaling are just a few of the proven modalities that help us to get our mind, body, and spirit in

sync. Cleansing your body and mind is very important, and it does take work.

9. Be a Kind Healer to Yourself. As I just wrote this, I chuckled to myself. I'm asking a Warrior class of people who would have died for the man next to them to be kind to themselves. And yet it is true: you need to be kind to yourself. Also, know that it's going to take work and time to learn to manage your PTS. Others have done it, and you can, too.

7

LIVING TO TELL

PLAIN common sense demands that doctors steer patients towards some other therapy than the zombie dope. We've had sixty years of benzos in society, and the sheer numbers of suicides and damaged minds and bodies show that as a clinical trial, that FDA approval back in the sixties has failed miserably. The maddening thing is that for the treatment of PTS, sleeplessness, anxiety, and depression, many other therapies work—and they don't poison people.

Of course, the baseline treatment for PTS and its symptoms is talk and behavioral therapy. Being around other Warfighters and opening up to each other about the bad thoughts and memories that trouble them can provide this service, too. So can journaling. Prayer works, too. The mind won't stop bringing up a problem until it's ad-

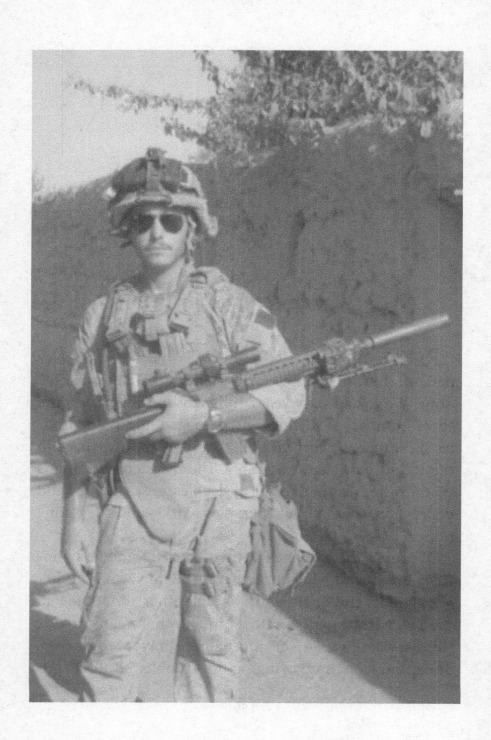

dressed. Doping the mind to make it shut up never fixes the original problem.

And beyond talking, other modalities offer a way to manage stress: yoga, Elohim's breathing, and meditation can all help. Beyond helping the mind, these ways of managing stress connect the mind to the body, which is so important. Bodies and minds affect each other in such intricate ways. One way to help the mind, too, is to improve the health of the body.

Cutting out sugar, caffeine, and alcohol can help the body rebalance itself. Though the transition away from junk food is hard, the rewards are worth all the trouble. The everyday American diet harms both the body and the mind, and sugar and caffeine alone can ramp up anxiety and paranoia even in civilians.

Want proof that sugar and caffeine mess you up? Go to a three-year-old kid's birthday party. Grownups are just like that, only instead of throwing a tantrum, they play video games for eight hours and pass out or go on an adrenaline-filled motorcycle ride and down a six-pack to calm the jitters.

Nobody needs to be on that hamster wheel.

Also, look at supplements and essential oils that can help with making the body feel at peace. I'm going to show you a ton of plants with no harmful side effects that can induce calm. You can find libraries worth of material on safe and gentle ways to treat anxiety, sleeplessness, and depression. And these ways won't come with a black-box warning.

First, let's look at the connection between mind and body.

"BREATH AND BODY"

Two therapy modalities that can help the body and inner self to heal one another are yoga and Elohim's breath. I put them together here because they both work in a similar way by unifying body and soul through paying attention to the breath. And as anyone can tell you, paying attention to the breath isn't going to put you at risk of suicide ideation.

That right there means that it's already miles ahead of whatever the pharmaceutical corporations have to offer.

"TRAUMA-CONSCIOUS YOGA"

I am a big believer in yoga! People all over the world use it daily to calm the mind and connect the body to the mind. It is so easy to go a day and not think about how deeply you're breathing and how your body really feels from the inside out. Best of all, we know that this practice stems from centuries of experience with no bad side effects.

The whole idea of yoga is that you use the pose of the body to increase mental awareness of it and connection to it. You let the peace of the mind flow into peacefulness in the body, and you let the natural energy in the body flow freely to every area. This goes against what we usually do.

When some area of the body is hurt, we coddle it; we shield it from getting any more trauma. But then our bodies tend to overuse the parts that are taking up the slack, causing more injury. The only way to bring healing to a long-injured part of the body is to give it the building blocks it needs to make new, healthy tissue and to work it gently to build its strength. Yoga is great for that!

Yoga can also work harmoniously with any faith practice. If your faith objects to the emptying of the mind many instructors teach, then you can fill your mind with religious texts like the Scriptures or with praise and worship music or prayer.

One of the best yoga practitioners I know personally is Judy Weaver, who co-founded Connected Warrior after helping a Warfighter with ALS remain strong and connected to his body while fighting the disease.[124] She very kindly wrote the following great section for me on Trauma-Conscious Yoga:

Trauma-Conscious Yoga is based on the understanding that trauma is held in the cells of the body and mind—it is physiological rather than psychological and that reconnecting the body and mind with the synchronization of conscious breath, movement and concentration in a safe, secure, and predictable environment supports healing and wellness. The evidence-based protocol manages and eases trauma's negative consequences occurring in the body and mind by reducing potential triggers of stress and providing choices, which is the opposite of trauma. Practitioners learn techniques to reconnect and develop awareness of the body and mind needs in that moment.

Social isolation is recognized as a primary contributing factor to suicide, and with 1 in 3 veterans suffering from a mental health diagnosis, suicide among past and present members of the military surpassed combat as a cause of death. Connected Warriors is directly battling our current suicide epidemic through work with trauma-conscious yoga instruction. A large part of the physical benefits is the release of calming and positive-thought-producing chemicals which occur when in social gatherings with like-minded individuals.

A multi-year study researching the effectiveness of trauma-conscious yoga instruction annotated additional physiological and psychological benefits, with participants reporting that one of the most meaningful outcomes was the camaraderie they experienced as a result of belonging to a group embracing yoga to improve their lives. Engagement in sessions helped participants to no longer feel isolated. (Nova Southeastern University) In July 2017, the American Journal of Preventive Medicine released a study by Dr. Erik J. Groessl and researchers from the VA San Diego Healthcare System on positive outcomes of our program. The study highlighted the improved behavioral-based pain management and a demonstrated decline in opiate use. In addition, a Connected Warriors-partnered scientific study operated in conjunction with the Department of Veterans Affairs found that

62% of participants reported positive reductions in pain, 70% increased levels of flexibility and balance, and 100% reported increased levels of social interaction and stress management behaviors.[125]

Connected Warriors partners with yoga studios to offer instruction to service members. But even if you can't find a studio near you, try yoga anyway. Try it at home with a free YouTube class if you want to learn the poses at home by yourself.

"What Is Elohim's Breath?"

You might remember the story of my back untwisting suddenly during a breathing session, unlocking the grief I'd been holding physically in my spine. That was a fireworks-level moment of revelation for me! My body knew how to do something that my mind was fighting, and I was suffering deeply and painfully because I wasn't letting the wisdom of my body heal my mind and soul.

We're so focused on the mind in Western societies. Ever since the Enlightenment freed us from being peasant slaves to superstition and poverty, we've all had the attitude: "Bring on the books, baby!" But in chasing knowledge, we've lost some other wisdom that we should take back.

In a similar way to yoga, Elohim's breath connects our minds and bodies. And I cannot tell you how much pain and trauma happens because our minds and bodies don't communicate well! It's like a troubled marriage—and Elohim's breath, which many who practice it still call transformational breath, is the couple's counseling that you need to get everybody talking again.

I asked Judith Kravitz to write something for me on this wonderful healing technique. She's an expert who has been practicing transformational breath since the seventies. People like Deepak Chopra and Christine Northrup recognize her incredible skill and profound knowledge.[126] Here's what she had to say:

Transformational Breath is a state-of-the-art system of breathing that works in multiple ways on each level of our being. Originating in the mid-70's through the inspiration of and development by Judith Kravitz, it has evolved in many ways over the four decades of growth and use.

Transformational Breath now shares its technique and programs in over 53 countries and remains the largest and fastest growing Breathing Modality in the world.

Beginning on the physical Level the overall intention is to open up the respiratory system so that the full use and capacity of the lungs is utilized and breathing becomes a conscious, safe and frequent practice. Most people do not consciously breathe, letting the autonomic nervous system kick in and unconsciously take a breath in that barely gives the many benefits that breath has to offer. Facilitators are trained to identify specific restricted breathing patterns then skillfully support and coach the client into a full, open, diaphragmatic breath. They also understand the behavioral and emotional patterns associated with each unique breathing pattern. Therefore by changing the patterns, behaviors and experiences change automatically.

Many major benefits happen on the physical level when breathing improves. More energy becomes available as the life force is enhanced by bringing in more air and oxygen and creating more space for breath in the body. Detoxification is greatly multiplied by the quick and relaxed exhale that is used. Cellular rejuvenation and nutrients are given through the expansion of the respiration and the oxygen rich blood. Major anaerobic conditions are eliminated by the increased overall oxygenation of the cells through improved daily breathing.

When the respiratory system is fully open it supports a balanced flow of not only energy but also balanced expression in life.

Since we have multiple levels of our being and they are all tied into each other, changes on one level create changes on all others. The opening of the respiratory system creates changes and integration on the mental, emotional, and spiritual level. In many ways what happens on those levels is a phenomenal mystery. While doing the Transformational Breath breathing pattern, which is initially through the mouth, using the diaphragm as the primary muscle, emphasizing the inhale and relaxing the exhale, with no pauses either between the inhale and exhale and the exhale and inhale, amazing things begin to happen. Especially breathing into areas that have traditionally been closed.

By consistently breathing in that way openly and fully some very interesting things begin to happen. It is very common when first breathing into a previously closed area, old memories and feelings can be accessed. These represent suppressed feelings, beliefs, and memories that were not able to be fully felt or expressed at the time of the experience. They are then pushed into the subconscious thus creating a vibrational filter which we experience life through. This filter prevents us from being fully present in the moment. Going through life we have layers and layers of these suppressed energetic filters that tend to distort our reality and affect how we either react or respond to our environment and experiences.

The high frequency energy from the TBr breathing pattern has the ability to access and then raise these lower frequency patterns in our energy field. This represents old feelings, memories, and negative thought patterns. This is quite amazing in that not only can we access the negativity in the subconscious but we have the opportunity to transform these lower energy patterns into a higher state. Therefore, this integrative work has the ability to tap into past traumas and memories at their core energetic state they exist on and change that frequency into a higher one. The end result is that negative thoughts and feelings that have been creating our life experiences are no longer resonating inside us the same way, so they are not attracting like energies and experiences in our life. In TBr not only can we breathe better and embody the many physical benefits, we can also free ourselves from cellular memories and feelings that would continue to out picture as unwanted, unpleasant experiences and feelings.

These first two levels we work on are really quite amazing and beneficial in themselves. Breathing better, living with improved

168

health and more vitality. Freeing the subconscious mind from mental and emotional patterns that keep us in unconscious bondage. However, the third level of TBr is the most profound. It is like the icing on the cake. Really good icing! We call it the spiritual level and the intention is to connect more deeply and live from our spiritual essence and nature. It is quite magical and also scientific as to how this happens. As the lower energy suppressions get raised to a higher vibrational state an opening is created to an expanded aspect of self. We get in touch with our innate love, peace, and joy, we can experience more awareness and higher consciousness states.

We are energetic beings, and the more we utilize this profound breathing tool the more open we become to our own higher nature. This expanded nature exists in each of us as our innate states of Peace, Love, and Joy.

The third level is ultimately the true intention of Transformational Breath, to connect more deeply and consciously with our spiritual nature. Yet first the breath needs to be fully present and free flowing in the body. Then the mental and emotional pieces that have been blocking the access to the higher subconscious have to be integrated to access the more refined aspects of ourselves. Each time we complete a TBr session the third level gets stronger and eventually we find ourselves enjoying life as the multidimensional being we are.[127]

There's an old Latin phrase that says: Dum spiro spero. It means, "While I breathe, I hope." People have always known the power of breath, which ties us to life and possibility and healing.

Warfighters know that pretending the enemy isn't there won't make him go away. They are trained to confront danger openly. This is why Elohim's breath is so great for them!

When Warfighters practice Elohim's breath, they invite the pain and grief and loss that are hiding in the shadows and conducting a radical guerilla warfare on the body and soul to come out into the open. Once those traumas step out of the shadows and into the light, Warfighters can deal with them as strong warriors.

Zombie dope is the soul equivalent of throwing a weapon aside and rocking on the floor. But Elohim's breath is like standing up, kicking a door down, and eliminating a threat once and for all. It's the path a Warfighter can and should take.

"THE WAY TO THE GYM"

My good friend Boone once told me that when you walk into the VA and ask the way to the pharmacy, everyone can give you directions. But when you walk into the VA and ask the way to the gym, no one knows where it is.

What kind of utter crap is that?

Look, before warfare, before trauma, Warfighters are elite athletes. Their bodies undergo a fierce transformation during boot camp and afterwards that enables them to do things ordinary humans can't. You read about the

Bataan Death March and the tough warriors who walked six days and nights without food, water, or rest, and you start to understand that military training makes a person into a different order of being than the common crowd.

A person like that has no business melting into a couch for days and weeks at a time. A person like that has no business letting those finely-tuned machines rust away. It's like fat Thor in the last Avengers: something about that picture just isn't right.

Move It or Lose It

Being a Warfighter is being a person who moves. Injuries happen, and bodies adjust. But I am constantly amazed at what a person's spirit can do when the body is limited. I see people running on blade-shaped prosthetics or playing basketball in souped-up wheelchairs, and I want to stand up and cheer.

Those people show us the greatest part of being human.

So, in encouraging a Warfighter to resume exercise, I'm not talking about refusing to acknowledge pain and limitation. Those things exist, and working around them is not easy. But exercise is like the super-drug that will improve nearly every area of life.

Doctors know this. That's why the first thing they tell almost everyone in an appointment is to eat right and exercise. They know that all the pills in the world can't do for you what moving around can do.

What can it do?

It gives you good sleep, improves digestion, regulates

mood swings, and pumps your body full of endorphins—natural happiness chemicals—all directly striking against symptoms of PTS like insomnia, stomach problems, anxiety, and depression. The Mayo Clinic lists seven benefits of exercise: weight control, fighting chronic diseases like diabetes and heart disease, improved mood, boost in energy, better sleep, increased sex drive, and mental health benefits of fun and social interaction.[128] And the Mayo Clinic is where you go if you're seriously ill. If anyone should know about how bodies work, it's them.

Doctors also say that exercise can help to prevent osteoporosis, stroke, and cancer. It can help us think more efficiently and make our skin look better. Hey, bonus! And it lowers our risk of depression and anxiety.[129]

Exercise reinforces goal setting. It increases strength and flexibility. It improves memory and self-confidence. It extends life.[130] It reduces stress and gets us out into nature, which is a whole other healing modality. It helps us battle addiction, become more creative, and get more done. It's a great well of inspiration and connection.[131]

Is it any wonder that exercise alone can act like a wonder drug? There is no doubt in the medical community or the alternative medicine community that exercise heals us. And because our bodies and minds are so connected, I know down to the last fiber of my being that a healthy, active body will do great things for the mind and soul, too.

"Warfighter Culture"

We all know, too, that being a Warfighter means that you are something more than an elite athlete. Sure, the military trains your body to do amazing things and to withstand incredible hardships. But it also conditions your soul and your mind into an identity that has more to do with Sparta and samurai than with ballers and sprinters.

Being a Warfighter goes beyond politics—beyond the divisions that strain America around election season. Warfighters aren't exclusively Republican or Democrat or Libertarian; they're not liberal or conservative. They're more than that.

Being a Warfighter means that you belong to a group, that you acknowledge a code, and that you prize others above yourself. It means that you're the wall against threat. It means that you are shaped by training and skill and ability to protect and defend.[132]

Being a Warfighter defines a state of mind. The warrior's mind is ready, prepared, tough, disciplined, and calm. The warrior's mind rises above wishes or despair to accept reality logically and proactively. A warrior's mind accepts no defeat, admits no surrender.[133]

Being a Warfighter changes the soul. A warrior's will disciplines his body and orders his mind. A warrior's inner being is capable of great focus, creativity, and decision. "Given enough time, any man may master the physical. With enough knowledge, any man may become wise. It is the true warrior who can master both....and surpass the result." (Tien T'ai)[134]

Warfighter culture stands on thousands of years of human history. It looks back to the traditions of the Assyrians, who used the latest technology and rigorous training to conquer the world of their time. It looks back to the Spartans, who disciplined themselves so thoroughly and prized honor so highly that three hundred of them could defeat an army of hundreds of thousands. It looks back to the Celts whose fearlessness and enthusiasm terrified Caesar. It looks back to the Roman legions, whose organization and determination won them an empire. It looks back to the sages of China and the samurai of Japan who created and recorded the philosophy of warfare. It uses all that is best and most praiseworthy from those who have learned the art of war to create new warriors.[135]

A warrior who returns home has to keep that mindset of warrior readiness, feeling useful and capable, not suffering the loss of self-esteem and confidence that someone sedentary suffers. Being a fighter, a winner, and a protector is an identity that exists deep inside a Warfighter. It's the reason a Warfighter fights wars in the first place.

A Warfighter has to remember who he or she is—and act on that.

"Walking Wounded"

People who return home from war suffer physical pain from wounds and from zombie dope. They suffer mental and emotional trauma from exposure to death and horror. They can't just act like everything is normal, like nothing happened. Expecting them to do so for the comfort and convenience of other people is beyond cruel.

So, what do you do with that real suffering? How do you begin to move forward in a limited body or a haunted soul? How do you both acknowledge what has happened in the past and step forward into the future?

That's a complicated question. But we have to try to answer it. So, let's look at three areas: physical injury, soul trauma, and coping mechanisms.

First, we'll look at physical injury. And I know that not all war wounds are immediately visible, like a lost limb or paralysis. I nursed Johnny through a bum knee and back; so I know how you can look fine from the outside but feel rotten. An injury is an injury.

So how do you keep going if you have an injury that causes you pain or limits the way your body works?

Some first steps are to accept your new reality and grieve what you've lost. You have to come to terms with what your body can do now. You are absolutely allowed to be pissed off at no longer having your former body. But you must settle into the life and physical form that belong to you now.[136]

Once you get a handle on the inner battle surrounding your physical reality, you can move on to practical steps. And let me just say here that I know that this is not just checking off items on a to-do list. Adjusting to a major physical life change like an injury is HARD. It SUCKS. There's no sugar coating how unfair and terrible it is. But here is the help I've found.

Some practical steps to take are to minimize the impact of daily life on your Warfighter. Arrange physical surroundings to make things as easy as possible for an injured person to be as independent as possible: ramps, toilet handles, lowered kitchen cabinets and counters. Find out what will help and do it. Use all the adaptive technology you can find. Put the injured person in charge of his or her own health as much as possible, and encourage making health a priority. Also, plug into a support network. No one can handle the transition to a new body without help.[137]

When it comes to daily living with a new physical reality, other people are so important. Though it's tempting to try to be strong and go it alone, interaction is the key to health. Think in terms of participation. Look at continuing education, finding a new hobby or activity, or volunteering.[138] Being of use to society can boost your mental health while you're adjusting to physical limitations. Bond with a pet—as far as I'm concerned, dogs are people, too!

Beyond physical injury, soul trauma is another hurdle for returning Warfighters. I saw in my beautiful son how depression, anxiety, and hard memories can put a person flat out on a couch as effectively as a physical injury. And often, the warrior culture that praises discipline and strength can make a Warfighter who is dealing with soul trauma feel embarrassed or guilty for not dealing with those inner demons.

I want to encourage everyone who loves a Warfighter to embrace this attitude of affirming capability. Battling those inner demons is one of the hardest fights a Warfighter will ever undertake. Taking even a small step towards life and hope is sometimes impossibly hard. Support those small steps and appreciate how much they cost.

Some of those small steps are really practical. One is to change things up. Go outside. Start something new. Make a schedule of healthy, life-affirming things to do, even if they're as simple as going for a walk or reading a book or playing with a kid. Discover or remember what floats your boat and go float it. Create rewards for sticking to the schedule. Reach for positive influences: positive people, positive music and media, and positive sources of encouragement, whether that comes from religion or philosophy.[139] Religion can provide immeasurable strength to those who are broken in spirit.

Another important step in moving forward with soul trauma is to get to know yourself really well. Understand your inner thoughts, desires, and weaknesses so that you can deal with the person you really are.[140] And something to consider deeply is that war may not be the root and foundation of your soul trauma.

Yep, we're going to talk about childhoods. Look, childhood lays everyone's foundation for adult life, and through absolutely no fault of your own, the adults in your life may have laid a really crappy foundation for you. So, when your soul slipped into the hell-brew that is combat, it didn't have the right tools to survive well.

There is no time like the present to look your kid self in the eye and acknowledge whatever did or didn't happen for you back then. Dealing with the past and repairing that crappy foundation is the way to build a really solid present. That shit isn't going away. Trust me.

And now that we've gotten cozy together talking about war trauma and rotten childhoods, we're going to go a step deeper and tackle depression, addiction, and coping mechanisms. Yeah, baby! Bring it on!

Depression, addiction, and coping mechanisms all feed into each other in a confusing and tenacious circle. When you feel bad (depression), you do something to make yourself feel better (coping mechanism), and sometimes that thing is not healthy. Do it enough, and you face addiction. But wait—addiction may exist as an inactive potential in your soul makeup, something that gets triggered when you're depressed. Experts don't know what causes what. And living with any of it is an exercise in frustration, patience, and persistence.[141]

Psychiatrists have found that about a third of the people dealing with depression also deal with addiction. They've also found a link between genetics and mental health, as well as a link between mental health and trauma and chemical changes to the brain. And they acknowledge that untreated depression and anxiety can lead to suicide.[142]

And you know by now what kind of chemicals Warfighters may have flooding through their systems—mefloquine, benzos, opioids, Agent Orange, and whatever nasty chemical cocktail Saddam Hussein left in the sand. Those chemicals cause real, physical changes to brain chemistry. If you're battling that kind of brain chemistry change on top of genetic inheritance, childhood damage, and combat trauma, then congratulations for getting out of bed this morning and breathing all day.

Seriously. Congratulations. I mean it. You're walking around with a two-hundred-pound rucksack all day, mentally and emotionally speaking, and that takes a lot of guts.

First of all, you should know that you're not alone. Around 1 in 5 Americans are dealing with some kind of mental illness like depression, anxiety, and addiction.[143] Second, you should know that there is hope. Healing of the mind and body is possible. And third and most important, you should know that healing comes through the simplest and hardest things.

Making a good food choice. Getting in fifteen minutes of exercise. Calling a friend. Taking a shower. Drinking water. See? Simple, but hard when all you want to do is check out with drink or sleep or drugs or other coping mechanisms.

What I desperately want to communicate to Warfighters and the people who love them is this. Physical and mental recovery is hard, but doable. And if anyone is cut out to do something hard, it's a Warfighter. So, take the condition of your body and the connection between your mind and body very seriously. Make it your job.

Because things can get better. And if you put that Warfighter mind and soul and will and body to the task, they will get better. Recognize, connect, and then live to tell your story.

"You Are What You Eat"

Nutrition in the military is largely a matter of getting enough calories in to fuel the war machine and getting those calories to Warfighters in a shelf-stable way that won't cause waste or disease. Nobody in Washington is designing a kale smoothie MRE. So, a Warfighter in active duty learns to eat a certain way: not picky.

The thing is that Warfighters can't eat the same way over here when they are not making the same demands on their bodies. And they shouldn't. We're talking about men and women who have been trained basically to be elite athletes in every way except nutrition. And part of the healing process is closing that gap and training War-fighters to fuel their human machines like the elite athletes that they are.

Making good choices in nutrition is as simple as following three basic rules. 1. No poisons, and by poisons I mean drugs, alcohol, and chemical additives to food. 2. Love water more than any other drink; your body needs it. And 3. Eat fresh food that will fuel your body instead of processed food that starves and fattens you at the same time.

RULE 1: NO POISONS

Let's start with the most obvious prohibition of all: illegal drugs. You guys have been getting this message since the fifth-grade "Just Say No" talk in health class, right? You've had people wagging fingers in your face for decades about illegal drugs.

But illegal drugs keep getting sold for two reasons. First, they work. They put you out so that you're not conscious of the things that bother you. Second, they're addictive. Start them, and you will have a fight on your hands to stop.

So, I'm going to tell you some facts about what they do to your body. And I'm not going to lie—facing those facts and doing the hard work of recovery will take all the willpower you have, along with a whole lot of help from friends, family, and professionals. But you need to use that willpower and lean on that community, because we all need you to live.

First, let's talk about what drugs do to your body. They come in three varieties: depressants, hallucinogens, and stimulants. Depressants slow your central nervous system. That may mean that you relax and lose your inhibitions or go to sleep, or it may mean that you stop breathing. You can't really pick once you get started.

Hallucinogens mean that you see things that aren't really there, or you feel extreme emotions like panic, paranoia, and euphoria. With the kinds of images and past emotions a Warfighter has tucked away, taking a hallucinogen is really a game of Russian roulette.

And stimulants speed up the central nervous system, causing sleeplessness, increased heart rate and blood pressure, anxiety, or seizures. They're a heart attack waiting to happen.[144]

The National CPR Association warns: "One of the possible effects of drug abuse is heart dysfunction, even in those who have no previous history of heart disease. A common side effect is arrhythmia, or an irregular heartbeat. Changes in blood pressure, heart attacks and stroke can occur when these drugs are taken in high doses. For those who already have a heart problem, illegal drug use may lead to worsening of their condition, and it can even lead to heart failure and death."[145]

One of the most dangerous things about illegal drugs

is that they're unpredictable. You can take a pill or a shot hoping to be relaxed, but you don't get to say how relaxed. Are you going to be relaxed enough to stop obsessing over bad memories, or are you going to be so relaxed that your central nervous system shuts down? You can reach for something to wake you up and make you feel again, but that something may make your heart race so fast it gives out. You may want something to give you happy dreams, but you don't get to pick what dreams come to you.[146]

So, besides the fact that these kinds of drugs can mimic or worsen some of the worst symptoms of PTS, which on its own is pretty crappy to do to a person, my HUGE problem with illegal drugs is that they take a person's choices away. Once you open yourself to them, they're in charge. They decide what you will do to get your next hit, and they decide how they'll affect you.[147]

I have to say that the rage monster inside me wakes up and starts yelling any time anyone gives up personal power. It makes me angry beyond words to know the way the government system takes advantage of the bravery and loyalty of Warfighters to experiment on them and give them doses of substances the service members don't know about. Fixing that problem is going to take a long time.

But hearing that Warfighters who have been lucky and blessed enough to survive combat or other trauma are VOLUNTARILY giving up control of their thoughts and actions and bodily functions to some chemical—that makes me red-hot mad.

Look—anyone who went through hell and back will need some help and hard work to heal. But checking out and handing your brain and body over to some chemical is not the answer. If that has happened to you or someone you love, it is not too late. You can come back and take control of your life again.

You can come back from any kind of addiction, and the next one we're going to talk about is addiction to alcohol. I have some room to talk here, because several years ago, I depended on alcohol to help me fall asleep and to forget my great loss. I was eating and drinking to die, not to live.

With help from friends and a health center, I learned a different way to live after loss. I learned that no amount of masking and hiding with any substance would take away the pain of loss. I would have to stay awake and aware and face that loss head on. I would have to reach out to Yahweh for strength and peace. And I learned truths about what the things I was taking in were doing to my body.

Here is what constant dependence on alcohol will do to your body, head to toe.

Starting with the head, it interrupts communication between your body and brain, affecting memory development and emotional control. Heavy drinkers are more likely to suffer heart disease. Alcohol inflames your pancreas, the organ your body uses to regulate your blood sugar. It destroys your liver, the organ your body uses to clean your blood. Alcohol abuse can lead to Type 2 diabetes from attacking these two organs. Drinking heavily damages the lining of your digestive tract, causing everything from diarrhea to malnutrition. Alcohol abuse leads to erectile dysfunction in men and to infertility in women, as well as hurting fetal development for pregnant women. Alcohol can weaken your bones, causing fractures and slowing their healing, and it can weaken your muscles and slow your immune system, making you more likely to catch everything from pneumonia and tuberculosis to the common cold.[148]

Medical studies prove a link between alcohol dependence and cancer.[149] Drinking a lot can give you seizures, arthritis, and infections.[150] It can lead to lapses in judgment, depression, and anxiety.[151] It can shrink your brain, contribute to dementia, and cause tremors.[152]

According to the CDC, "Excessive alcohol use led to approximately 88,000 deaths and 2.5 million years of potential life lost (YPLL) each year in the United States from 2006 to 2010, shortening the lives of those who died by an average of 30 years. Further, excessive drinking was responsible for 1 in 10 deaths among working-age adults aged 20-64 years. The economic costs of excessive alcohol consumption in 2010 were estimated at $249 billion."[153]

I could go on—trust me—but after reading all of those facts, you have to see that the risks of heavy drinking just aren't worth any kind of reward. I have found other ways to heal the pain inside me, and I promise you that you can, too. Any Warfighter has enough to do healing from injury and grief without heaping all of those bad health consequences on top of it. Addiction to alcohol will only make things worse, and it could take your life.

If you're going to *Live to Tell* your story, first you have to live.

The final part of the no poisons rule is food chemicals. This is a sneaky one. You may feel pretty good about yourself so far because you don't abuse alcohol or drugs. But those TV dinners, cheese puffs, and packaged cupcakes are doing a heck of a lot of damage, too.

The most common types of food additives are food dyes. But even though these chemicals are approved by the FDA, they cause problems like hyperactivity and asthma. The FDA removed one red dye back in the 1970s because it caused cancer in rats. Also not great are preservatives like sodium benzoate and sodium nitrites. Sodium benzoate can cause hyperactivity, and with added vitamin C, it can produce benzene, which causes cancer. Sodium nitrites have been linked to gastric cancer.[154]

Artificial flavors can cause allergy symptoms or behavior problems; olestra, an artificial fat, can cause stomach and intestine trouble. All the excess salt in prepackaged foods can cause you to retain fluid or develop high blood pressure. And the kind of refined and processed flour used in factory bakeries has low nutrition and, with the wheat bran and germ removed, can affect insulin.[155]

We really have to watch for sugars, too, both natural and substitutes. With the rates of obesity and diabetes soaring, doctors are constantly beating the no-sugar drum, but honestly, some of the fake sugars can be dangerous, too. Aspartame is a nerve poison and cancer contributor that can cause "brain tumor, diseases like lymphoma, diabetes, multiple sclerosis, Parkinson's, Alzheimer's, fibromyalgia, and chronic fatigue, emotional disorders like depression and anxiety attacks, dizziness, headaches, nausea, mental confusion, migraines and seizures." And high fructose corn syrup, which is sugar under another name, contributes to weight gain, "increases your LDL ("bad") cholesterol levels, and contributes to the development of diabetes and tissue damage, among other harmful effects."[156]

Methylcyclopropene is a gas sprayed on apples and bananas to keep them from rotting. BHA and BHT, derived from petroleum, are chemicals used to preserve food; they cause cancer. Canthaxanthin, used to make egg yolks look more yellow, can cause retinal damage.[157]

Transfats can cause inflammation, heart disease, and diabetes. Yeast extract and MSG can cause headaches, swelling, numbness, and gastrointestinal distress to people who are sensitive to them.[158] Even plastic and paper food packaging contains chemicals like bisphenols, phthalates, perfluoroalkyl chemicals, and perchlorate that can cause problems with fertility, the thyroid, the immune system, the cardiovascular system, and the nervous system.[159]

There are so many more chemicals to watch for. I would have to write a whole book on them to list them and their side effects! When it comes down to it, you should know that food companies are not required to get prior approval from the FDA before using a food chemical. The FDA relies on the corporate food industry to police itself! This has resulted in over 10,000 chemicals being used in different combinations in our food. And studies show that these chemicals are much more dangerous in combination.[160]

Warfighters in active service don't have much control over what goes into their bodies, especially during deployment. That's why it's so important to pay attention to things like food chemicals. The more you know, the more control you have over your health. If you or a Warfighter you love is suffering symptoms of PTS, why pile on the extra digestive and nerve problems that food chemicals can cause?

Cutting out corporate food is just eliminating one more battle you don't have to fight.

RULE 2: LOVE WATER

We've just covered a lot of different kinds of poisons that can accumulate in your body. And we haven't even mentioned air pollution and the toxic chemicals that have accumulated in the ground and water. This is one reason why drinking enough water is such an important part of a healing strategy.

Our bodies are composed of a high percentage of water—I've seen statistics between 60 and 90 percent—and every kind of fluid inside us needs water to do its job well. This means your blood, every hormone, and most importantly, waste removal. Your kidneys can get rid of a whole lot of poisons if they have enough water to work with.[161]

And staying hydrated can help you stay at peak performance. We talked a lot about the importance of exercise, what a miracle drug that is. Well, losing even 2% of your body's water content can keep you from performing at your peak. And it's not just your body. Being dehydrated can affect your brain function, like mood and concentration. A great way to stay at your best is to stay hydrated.[162]

Adequate water can help you keep from getting sick. It can fight hangovers, and it can keep you from being constipated. It banishes fatigue and can help with weight loss. A lot of times, when people think they're hungry, they're really just thirsty.[163]

Water can prevent and relieve headaches, which are often caused by dehydration. It also keeps joints and muscles elastic and moving well so that you are less likely to cramp up or get a sprain. And though I'm not saying anybody's vain, it does help skin look clear and healthy![164]

Here is a cool thing water can do—regulate body temperature. If you have enough water in your system, your body can sweat—to cool you off. If you don't, you can't tolerate the heat as well. Cool, huh? And besides that, water cushions your brain, spinal cord, and other sensitive tissues. Also, did you know that it helps your lungs? If you're not hydrated, your body restricts your airways in an attempt to minimize water loss, which can worsen problems like asthma and allergies.[165]

Bottom line—being hydrated will make everything else so much easier. It will help with literally every health condition, because every part of your body needs enough water. If you are hydrated, you will feel better and be able to do more.

RULE 3: EAT FRESH

When I talk about eating fresh foods, I'm talking about breaking the MRE mindset. I'm talking about steering clear of the foods you grab because they're easy or to treat yourself. Eating that way exposes you to a lot of food chemicals and additives, and it robs your body of a lot of good stuff like vitamins and proteins and enough water.

If you eat fresh foods, you won't have to think about reading labels and researching fourteen-syllable chemical names to see what they are and if they're going to kill you in ten years. It's just easier that way.

It's harder in another way. If you choose to start eating real, fresh food, then you or someone you love is going to have to put in some time shopping, prepping, and cooking. There's a lot more washing, chopping, and peeling involved in eating real food.

But boy, is it worth the trouble!

Produce loses its nutritional value quickly. So, you have to eat it pretty close to when it's picked to get the nutritional value. Eating fresh means that you're getting the most from your food.[166]

Eating fresh food makes sure that your body has what it needs to keep you going. You need antioxidants to make up for the wear and tear on your system. You need proteins to repair the normal damage from using your muscles. You need water and the proper amounts of sodium and vitamins, all of which you can get from healthy food. If you eat well, you're more likely to stay in a healthy weight range, which will lower your risk of disease.[167]

Eating vegetables and fruits in particular does wonderful things for your body. It lowers your risk of heart disease, diabetes, and cancer. It ups your intake of things like fiber and water that lower your blood cholesterol and keep you regular, and therefore reduce your chance of getting colon cancer. Potassium regulates blood pressure. Folate helps in making red blood cells, oxygen carriers. Getting enough vitamins and other nutrients prevents disease.[168]

Eating healthy means eating a good balance of different kinds of things. The Harvard Healthy Eating Pyramid includes all of these varied nutrients. "While some extreme diets may suggest otherwise, we all need a balance of protein, fat, carbohydrates, fiber, vitamins, and minerals in our diets to sustain a healthy body. You don't need to eliminate certain categories of food from your diet, but rather select the healthiest options from each category."[169]

We now know about specific benefits from specific types of food; so we can shop the grocery store for specific health benefits. As Hippocrates said, "Let food be thy medicine and medicine thy food."[170] We can do that more specifically now than ol' Hippocrates ever dreamed.

Oats can lower cholesterol, help with weight loss, and improve the skin. Wild salmon can reduce belly fat, lower cholesterol, and fight sun damage, reducing precancerous skin lesions. A Harvard study showed that eating blueberries and strawberries three times a week cut heart attack risk in women by 30 percent. Avocados help with weight loss and metabolic syndrome. Walnuts benefit the heart and are full of protein and fiber.[171]

Beef is loaded with iron, while chicken is low in fat but high in protein. So are shrimp and tuna. Garlic boosts the immune system. Brown rice provides fiber, vitamin B1, and magnesium. Lentils are high in protein and fiber. Yogurt is high in protein, and its natural probiotics do wonderful things for your gut. Coconut oil can help with Alzheimer's disease. Dark chocolate provides magnesium and antioxidants.[172]

And look, we all want to eat food that looks and tastes good. And we are much more likely to eat well if we're eating what tastes good. Prepackaged food has to do a lot of chemical gymnastics to add back the color and flavor and texture of foods that they have processed all the goodness out of. Fresh food just tastes good already. It has a greater variety of colors, textures, and flavors than processed foods do.[173]

Taking the time to eat well is one of the best things you can do for yourself. And if you take care of yourself by following the three rules: no poisons, love water, and eat fresh, then you will definitely see a benefit. Team up the three rules with exercise, yoga, and Elohim's breath, and you will be amazed at how your body responds.

Plants, not Poisons

When you go to the VA with PTS symptoms, you're looking for a specific kind of relief. You are probably experiencing the insomnia, depression, anxiety, and pain that are the most common symptoms. The relief that the VA is going to offer you comes with a trade-off—lots of appalling side effects that will require even more medication, which will cause even more side effects. I want to stop that nasty cycle from ever starting.

In the same way that certain foods provide certain benefits, certain herbs provide certain benefits. They can help you sleep, lift your depression, calm your anxiety, and treat your physical pain. And those benefits won't come with a complicated trade-off. They'll just help, without hurting at the same time.

One caution—some of these herbs can react with prescription medication. So, if you're taking a prescription, check with your doctor to make sure that the herbs you want to take won't cancel out or exaggerate the effects of the prescription.

You may find the same herb under multiple sections, because many of these herbs do more than one thing. One plant may boost your mood, help you sleep, and calm your anxiety, all at once. Bonus!

Interested? Read on.

"For Good Sleep"

Before we get started with the herbal supplements, here are some natural remedies to help you sleep. Inversion, or at least elevating your feet above your heart, can reduce swelling and inflammation and redistribute the lymph that's pooled in your lower body throughout the day. You can also try a combination of half a teaspoon of honey and a sprinkle of salt at least fifteen minutes before going to bed. Cherry juice can reduce inflammation and raise melatonin for a good insomnia treatment. Deep breathing and daily exercise also help.[174]

Also, try light therapy during the day. Getting light in the day can help regulate your sleep cycles at night. Meditation and gentle yoga stretching can prepare your mind and body to sleep. If you're feeling adventurous, acupuncture or hypnosis may help. Or try listening to slow, gentle music.[175] After a recent trip that knocked me off kilter for a while, I started listening to thunderstorms and sleep stories on YouTube. They kept my mind occupied lightly so that I could rest.

"On to the Herbs!"

Passionflower helps relieve anxiety and calm nerves, and it can soothe restless leg syndrome. California poppy relieves anxiety, stress, and pain. Hops, the same plant used to make beer, will relieve anxiety and restlessness and help you stay asleep longer once you get to sleep. Chamomile is a mild sedative that also helps soothe stomach troubles. Lavender decreases anxiety and insomnia and helps you fall into a deeper sleep that leaves you feeling better in the morning.[176]

Valerian root relieves insomnia and depression, and it can help you fall asleep faster. Lemon balm calms you, helping with anxiety, depression, and sleep problems. It also helps with digestive issues.[177]

Kava makes you feel sleepy and calm. St. John's Wort helps with anxiety, depression, and sleeplessness. Interestingly, it bonds naturally to the same GABA receptors that benzodiazepines affect, but without the negative effects.[178]

Magnesium and calcium promote sleep, especially taken together. Wild lettuce can treat anxiety, headaches, muscle and joint pain, and restless leg syndrome. Melatonin is the hormone that controls sleep; taking it at a low dose will help insomnia.[179]

"FOR A BRIGHTER MOOD"

When you have depression, your symptoms go beyond just feeling sad. You feel hopeless and lost. You can't muster the energy for the simplest tasks. Showering and brushing your teeth seem like climbing a mountain.

I know what that feels like. And none of these supplements alone are going to cure that kind of heavy depression. What I'm suggesting are helps to use along with other treatments like talk therapy, mind-body connection through yoga and Elohim's breathing, improved diet and exercise, and time with supportive people and animals.

Again, make sure to check with your doctor for interactions with prescription medication. No one approach is going to clear the fog surrounding you. But the modalities I've found can be part of that treatment.

And unlike zombie dope, these modalities won't steal your mind, your time, or your life.

First on the list is our old friend St. John's Wort, which also works on insomnia and anxiety. Saffron, the spice that gives Spanish rice and paella its color, can help with depression. SAM-e, which stands for S-adenosylmethionine, acts like your body's own natural mood-lifting chemicals. Also eat fish or take Omega-3 oils; the Mayo Clinic found that a deficiency in these oils can lead to depression. So can a lack of folate; so take folic acid or eat foods like "beans, lentils, fortified cereals, dark leafy greens, sunflower seeds, and avocados." Low levels of zinc in the blood are linked to depression, too, so take a supplement.[180]

5-HTP, which we listed for anxiety, is a synthetic tryptophan. It works on depression. Vitamin B6 helps your body make serotonin and dopamine. Magnesium helps produce serotonin, too.[181] Your body makes the hormone DHEA; changes in its levels have been linked to depression. Yu may want to take a synthetic DHEA under a doctor's supervision.[182]

Speaking of treatments to try under a doctor's supervision, your depression may have its root in a hormone imbalance. Low testosterone or estrogen can mess with your mood like you wouldn't believe! Other hormones, too, can cause depression when they're not balanced. You can have a doctor run the following tests and help you develop a balancing treatment plan:

Thyroid gland tests – TSH, free T4, free T3, total T3, thyroid antibodies

Adrenal gland tests – cortisol, DHEA-S, pregnenolone

Sex hormone tests – estradiol, progesterone, free and total testosterone[183]

As with anxiety, some treatments are behavior based. This is where having support from friends and family will come in handy. Some of these suggestions will seem beyond your ability even to consider. You will need the help of a friend to pull you into them.

Of course, maintaining your physical health is so important. Exercise, water, clean food, meditation, and sleep are so important for treating depression. A happy mind has a harder time taking up residence in a sick body. In addition to staying healthy, getting out into nature can help lift depression. Bright sunlight also helps.[184]

Also helpful are getting into a routine and setting goals. They can help you find a sense of purpose and sanity that can draw you back into life. Speaking of purpose, take on some responsibility. Start small. But your depressed self will want to withdraw from everything; we want to counteract that tendency. And challenge your thinking. Dark thoughts will come to you, but you can question them instead of accepting them as true. Try new things. Try to have fun.[185]

You can see pretty quickly that you're going to need a loved one to help you want to do some of these things. Community is so important in treating depression, especially in the Warfighter community. Look at it this way.

When you were trained to fight, you were trained to work as a unit with other people. Even elite warriors like Rangers and SEALs learn to work as a team. Use what was effective in one kind of combat to fight this battle against the darkness.

Your buddies were there for you then. Buddies can be there for you now. They're a proven resource in the battles at home.

"For a Calmer Mind"

Anxiety is debilitating. It brings worry over the past together with dread of the future to make your present unlivable. That's why VA doctors bring out the big guns to treat it—the zombie dope. But you can get a calming effect without missing out on your life or running the other risks associated with benzos and opioids.

Kava physically calms you down, treating muscle spasms and tension and making you feel sleepy and relaxed. It also helps soothe anxious thoughts. Lemon balm helps with stress and anxiety: "in one study of healthy volunteers, a daily dose of 600 mgs of lemon balm for a week improved mood, and boosted both calmness and alertness." Theanine from green tea relieves stress. Valerian makes you feel serene and calm. The scent of lavender produces calm. And chamomile calms and relaxes your body and mind.[186]

Ginger can relieve stress, among its other benefits like headache and stomachache relief. Ginseng improves brain circulation and reduces inflammation; it helps with both anxiety and depression. Ashwagandha, also known as Indian Ginseng, provides anti-anxiety benefits. Ginkgo biloba lifts the mood, calms the mind, and relieves anxiety. St. John's Wort treats anxiety and depression. Omega-3 oils, sold in supplements and also available in food like fish and walnuts, relieves anxiety in addition to promoting a healthy heart. And passionflower helps not just insomnia but anxiety: "One study involving people with generalized anxiety disorder found that taking passion flower drops helped to manage anxiety. When compared with benzodiazepine drugs, passionflower supplements were just as effective for anxiety without many of the side effects."[187]

A synthetic form of tryptophan, 5-HTP, treats insomnia, mood swings, and headache pain. GABA supplements help with anxiety, sleeplessness, ADHD, PMS, blood pressure, and pain relief. B vitamins help with regulating moods, stabilizing blood sugar, and soothing the nervous system, especially B6 and B12.[188]

Arctic root strengthens the body's physical and mental reaction to stress. Bacopa promotes memory and attention while relieving stress. Vitamin D boosts mood and relieves stress; you can get outside in the sun or take a supplement. Taurine works with GABA receptors to do the same job a benzo tries to do. Because your gut is your second brain, affecting mood and brain activity, taking a probiotic to improve gut health can relieve anxiety. Gotu kola tea is traditional in Chinese medicine, which recommends it for "disorders of the mind including anxiety, mental fatigue, depression, memory loss, and insomnia." Tea made from tulsi, or holy basil, can help reduce cortisol. Argentum nitricum, derived from silver nitrate, calms anxious thoughts. Aconitum napellus, also known as monkshood or wolf's bane, works with sudden anxiety and panic. Essential oils can also help: "Bergamot essential oil has been shown to [be] similarly effective for anxiety as the anti-anxiety drug Valium. Other essential oils to consider for anxiety include rose, neroli, sandalwood, ylang-ylang, geranium, and jasmine."[189]

In addition to these supplements, the food you eat may help you calm your anxious thoughts. A field called nutritional psychiatry makes these correlations between nutrients and mind health. Tuna, salmon, walnuts, and flaxseed all provide Omega-3 oils, which alleviate anxiety. L-lysine and L-arginine found in foods like cheese, red meat, and fish reduce anxiety symptoms. Get plenty of magnesium, vitamin B12, and zinc. Blueberries and peaches can relieve stress. Whole grains and oats produce serotonin, a happiness hormone. You can lower the stress hormone cortisol by eating citrus, leafy greens, and dark chocolate.[190]

Besides supplements and food, behavior strategies can help with treating anxiety. Exercise, therapy, and meditation you already know. Writing can help a great deal; I've found journaling a good stress relief. Creative writing helps, too. Time management tools like calendars and planners can help organize and manage stresses and time commitments to make life seem more doable. And spending time with animals helps, too. Even caring for crickets reduces anxiety. Specifically, caring for horses seems to alleviate trauma-related stress.[191] Those cowboys were onto something!

"For Pain Relief"

This is the big problem, because if your body is suffering pain, you won't be able to get sleep. You'll suffer anxiety about the pain, and the sleeplessness and anxiety will cause depression. I remember what my back felt like when my body was storing grief there. I remember what it was like to feel so much pain that I was caught like a rabbit in a trap - willing to chew something off to get free.

But if you can strike a blow here and treat the chronic pain without dangerous pharmaceuticals, you will be well on your way to getting better. Feeling good in your body puts you one step closer to feeling good in your mind and soul. Remember, all of these treatments work together: food, water, exercise, therapy, supplements, and proactive choices toward life, like friendship and connection to animals and nature.

As far as things you can take, you can use willow bark, the plant source for aspirin. Some help is as close as your spice cabinet: turmeric and cloves can both help with pain relief. And besides those substances, you may find relief with acupuncture, which has been proven to release serotonin, and from the application of heat and cold.[192]

Chiropractic care, whether through massage or adjustment, can help align bones and muscles to relieve pain. If you can stand it, stretching and exercise will release endorphins, which can relieve pain. And believe it or not, simply going barefoot outside can transfer free electrons from the earth, which can relieve inflammation.[193]

Two techniques of mindfulness may help. One is zooming in, focusing on the area of the body that is in pain. Only instead of just pain, you're encouraged to note other sensations, like tightness, tingling, or pulling. This mindfulness can remove the emotional associations of pain. The other technique is zooming out, where you're encouraged to focus on other areas of the body that are not in pain. Gradually you move outward from your body to spread your attention to gratitude and other positive emotions.[194]

Here's another radical idea: cryotherapy or cold exposure. Intense cold can reduce inflammation and release specific proteins in the body that speed healing. Meditation and mindfulness do an amazing job relieving pain and helping you bear it. Back to things you can take as a supplement, Boswellia or frankincense reduces inflammation and specifically helps the joints. MSM or Methylsulfonylmethane is a potent antioxidant that reduces inflammation, especially in the joints.[195]

Another supplement to take is resveratrol, a substance occurring naturally in grapes and berries. It heals the body at a cellular level, and it relieves pain. And if cold therapy doesn't work for you, you may want to try heat therapy. Immersion in warm water, especially with the additions of Epsom salts and massage, can help the pain.[196]

More herbs used for many years to treat pain are skullcap, which treats pain and anxiety; feverfew, which treats toothaches, headaches, and stomachaches; and devil's claw, which treats lower back pain and arthritis.[197]

Capsaicin from chili peppers can help pain when applied to the skin. Glucosamine can help with arthritis pain. Modalities like yoga, relaxation therapy, hypnosis, guided imagery, music therapy, biofeedback, and massage can all help relieve pain. Not everyone is the same - you have to find what works for you.[198]

"Cannabis"

One incredibly helpful therapy that's becoming increasingly available as state legislatures become more educated is cannabis and its non-hallucinogenic derivative, CBD oil. Throughout the 1800s, doctors used and prescribed cannabis, calling it by its Latin name. In 1937, the government passed the Marijuana Tax Act, and those who were arrested for illegal sale were arrested for tax violations. In 1952, the Boggs Act required sentencing for drug-related convictions. Cannabis did not become illegal until the Controlled Substances Act of 1970.[199]

People who immediately object to this therapy are most likely responding to rhetoric born in the twenties and thirties. Prohibition-era government agents pled their case against cannabis, newly labeled marijuana to make it seem more Hispanic and threatening,[200] in racially charged newspapers—newspapers that were discussing the "yellow peril" and the "Negro problem" on the same pages as "reefer madness" and condemning everyone from Mexican refugees to Hindu immigrants to black jazz musicians for corrupting whites with the stuff.[201]

Today, more and more people are realizing the racially and culturally motivated nature of the laws against cannabis and discovering the disproportionate arrests and sentencing of minorities under these laws. More people every day are working to change state and federal laws to reflect the reality of what the cannabis plant is and what it can do. Even Harvard Medical School admits the effectiveness of medical marijuana and especially CBD in managing chronic pain and tremors, among other symptoms.[202]

However, doctors still have misgivings. An article in the *Journal of the American Medical Association* notes multiple risks and benefits of medical marijuana. It admits effectiveness in randomized clinical trials on chronic pain and tremors associated with diseases like Parkinson's, epilepsy, and multiple sclerosis. It notes that smoked marijuana has more pharmacologically active compounds than the current FDA approved cannabis-derived medications.

Then it makes this statement: "According to the US government, marijuana is an illegal drug that is classified as Schedule I under the Controlled Substances Act, meaning that it has no currently accepted medical use and a high potential for abuse. Marijuana's status as a Schedule I substance that is illegal according to the federal government is the reason that physicians cannot prescribe medical marijuana and can only certify its use."[203]

The position of the federal government against cannabis is only one factor in the attitude of doctors. One 2013 Colorado survey reported in the *Journal of the American Board of Family Medicine* details the reluctance of family physicians to prescribe marijuana in that state, where it had been legal for medical use since 2000. The two biggest factors in whether a doctor would prescribe marijuana for a patient qualified by law to need it were 1) experience with patients and 2) medical literature.[204]

This conclusion shows the never-ending cycle of marijuana opposition. Doctors would be more likely to prescribe or certify marijuana if it appeared favorably in the medical literature; if they had personal experience using it in treatment with patients; and if they had no concerns about legal repercussions for them, their patients, and their practices. However, as long as marijuana remains illegal federally, they will not prescribe or certify it for patients, and they will be less likely to conduct and organize funding for the kind of randomized, clinical trials on medical marijuana use that can then appear in peer-reviewed medical literature.

Clearly, federal opposition is damaging the doctor-patient relationship and the well-being of patients. And this cycle will only change direction when the federal government allows it to change by descheduling marijuana as not a Schedule 1 drug like heroin or ecstasy.[205] So it's up to we the people to tell the federal government we've had enough. And yes, we want it descheduled, not rescheduled. We want to keep it in the hands of the local dispensaries and out the hands of the pharmaceutical companies.

Until the government hears us, there's CBD.

CBD is one of 120 compounds found in marijuana. CBD oil available commercially is made of this one compound isolated and mixed with a neutral oil like coconut oil or olive oil. Industrial hemp, a related plant, has higher levels of CBD; therefore, most CBD oil comes from hemp instead of marijuana. CBD does not contain THC, the compound in marijuana that causes hallucinations and loss of motor control. So, taking CBD does not make you high like you see in the stoner movies.[206] And according to the World Health Organization, CBD is not addictive.[207]

Scientific evidence backs six major benefits of CBD oil: 1) pain relief, 2) reduced anxiety and depression, 3) relief of nausea and vomiting, 4) treatment of acne, 5) calming of seizures, and 6) lowering of high blood pressure. In addition, studies show that CBD may also alleviate mental disorders, slow tumor growth, help recovering addicts, and treat diabetes.[208] And unlike benzos and opioids, CBD does not damage the kidneys, irritate the stomach lining, or cause life-threatening side effects like suicide ideation.

Unfortunately, CBD is not legal in all 50 states. It's currently legal in the 30 states that already allow medical cannabis. "Seventeen additional states have CBD-specific laws on the books, according to Prevention magazine. Those are Alabama, Georgia, Indiana, Iowa, Kentucky, Mississippi, Missouri, North Carolina, Oklahoma, South Carolina, South Dakota, Tennessee, Texas, Utah, Virginia, Wisconsin and Wyoming."[209] The article that talks about legality also advocates regulation, expressing concerns that unregulated products may not contain what they say they do.

My friend, prominent veteran advocate Boone Cutler, makes the case for medical marijuana and CBD specifically for veterans because of the drugs that military service exposes them to. "It does the opposite of what the Mefloquine does. Mefloquine takes away your impulse control. So, if you have an impulse to commit suicide, you are likely to do it without thinking. Medical marijuana fights that impulse. If a guy is not doing well and he takes benzos, he's going to battle suicide ideation on top of the mefloquine toxicity, and the outlook is not good. But what's the worst that can happen if he takes CBD, or if he smokes a joint? He gets distracted from that impulse and falls asleep. When he wakes up, he doesn't have that impulse. Sounds a whole lot better and safer to me."[210]

And I can tell you without a doubt that if my son had been allowed and advised to take CBD for his sleeplessness and anxiety instead of the dangerous benzodiazepines he was prescribed and expected to take, he would be alive today. You can talk about the pros and cons and how many clinical trials and medical articles there are all you want, but the difference is clear.

Benzos rob Warfighters of their independence. CBD does not. Benzos are deadly. CBD is not. We owe it to patients across America as a whole but to veterans especially to give them the pain and anxiety relief option that is not deadly.

It is truly a matter of life and death.

"THE VERY BEST BUTTER"

I remember watching Alice in Wonderland with my kids at daycare. Do you remember the scene where the watch breaks, and the cuckoo bananas Mad Hatter and March Hare smear the gears and springs inside with butter? When Alice objects, they tell her that they're only using the very best butter.

You're not supposed to put butter inside a watch. Anyone knows this. It's not a fix that has any hope of working.

I can't stress this enough. Elohim has made our bodies to run well in this world if they have the materials they need, like food, sleep, exercise, and water. Supplying the body is like winding the watch. And when something goes wrong, like trauma or injury, it's like dust in the gears. The natural healing modalities and supplements we've discussed are like cleaning the gears and oiling them to run smoothly.

Demanding prescription medication for emotional trauma is like smearing the gears with the very best butter. It's not working with the machine in the way it was designed to operate. People think of natural remedies as some way-out, experimental voodoo.

What's way out there and experimental is the zombie dope that has been circulating for a tiny fraction of time, compared to natural remedies. And the evidence of real people losing their lives by non-participation or suicide is enough to show that the corporate medicine experiment is a huge mistake. It's time to stop using our veterans like lab rats and get back to what people all over the world have known for years will work. It's time to stop selling the American taxpayer the very best butter.

8

LIVE TO TELL

IN coming to the end of *Live to Tell*, I know that I have to include a very painful part of my family story, one I haven't known how to mention before now. This book is about veteran suicide, and I want to focus on that problem and what the death of my son Johnny forced me to learn about it. So I've kept to the story of Johnny's military service, his transition home, his battle with zombie dope, and his death by pharmaceutical induced suicide.

I want to do right by my son Johnny. I want people to know his story, and I want people who love veterans to know how to keep his story from becoming theirs. So *Live to Tell* is rightfully Johnny's book.

But I have two sons.

Justin, my younger sweet son, was the person who found Johnny's body.

I will never know the depth of the trauma that Justin

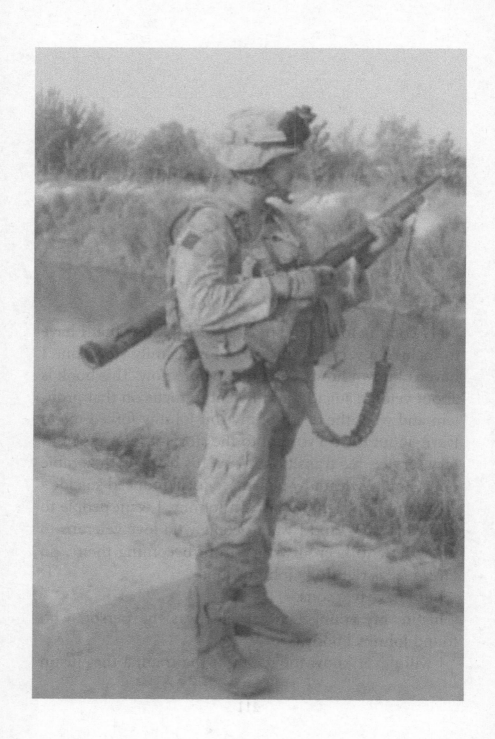

endured in that moment. I will never know the permanent scarring that finding Johnny inflicted on his soul. All I know for sure is that Johnny's loss stayed with Justin. It hurt him and kept hurting him.

The two boys had always been close. I had kept them with me while I worked and let them run all around Super Stone together. They were each other's first friends and playmates.

I found a letter the other day that Justin wrote to Johnny when he was deployed. I had let my ex-husband come over to stay for the holidays, as I did sometimes, and he had just left. So, a fifteen-year-old-Justin wrote to Johnny:

Homedog—

What up, home skillet? Not much has changed around here except for the fact that dad left. Well, I love and miss you so much. Love you, Johnny,

Love, Justin (Homedog)

Eight months after Johnny's death, Justin moved to Orlando, because he had friends there. Justin got a job with Comcast. They called Super Stone for a job recommendation. And of course, we gave him an outstanding one. We couldn't say enough good things about him. So, he got the job.

213

Soon afterwards, he told me that he wanted to come back home, work with the company, and go to school. I was so happy. He also asked to see a psychiatrist.

I was going to counseling at the vet center. I told the director there, Jeff Flowers, what Justin had said about wanting to see a psychiatrist. Jeff said, "Janine, you need to do that immediately." I planned to do so as soon as Justin came home. Then he just stopped responding to me.

As I later discovered, Justin wrote a goodbye note on his phone, deleted all previous messages from everybody, and he killed himself.

People have asked me how I could bear such a tragedy not once but twice. At times in my life, I have been sure that I could not bear it. I have thought of following my boys through the same door that claimed them.

I know now that Elohim was watching over me to keep me safe. He's the reason I'm still here. He's that little voice that whispered in my ear, you know, 'Hey, maybe if you cleared your mind, you could think of another way to live.'"

Everything good, everything good comes from him. You know? The tragedies that happen in our life, I don't understand why they happen. But my children were adult children, and they made those decisions.

And how blessed I was to have them for the twenty-four years I had them! You know? They were a blessing to me. I can be grateful for that time.

If I can get across one main thought, it's this. Suicide

doesn't get rid of pain. It just spreads it around to everyone who loves you.

I get it. People who have suicidal thoughts are just in so much pain inside, and they think that they're better off dead. When they get to the point that they're in that much pain, they can't see beyond it.

All I can say, from the depths of my heart, is that you don't know the effect you have on other people's lives. You can't predict the ripple effect of suicide. You can't control that transference of pain.

I'm sure Johnny didn't realize how much pain his death would cause Justin. I'm sure Johnny didn't want that. He wanted Justin to live. He wanted him to be happy, to have a better relationship with me, to be healthy and lose weight and date cute chicks. That's what my Marine son with his good heart wanted.

And we who love veterans have got to wake up and realize that our veterans aren't choosing this way of death. This is not them. This is not who they are or what they want.

They are battling the effects of drugs like Mefloquine given to them dishonestly.

They are battling zombie dope that kills their capacity for joy and independence and fills them with thoughts of death.

They are battling a system that treats them with an alarming lack of respect for the sacrifices they have made and the dangers they face at home.

They are battling separation from the only community that understands them and means anything to them.

They are battling a lack of knowledge about the true nature of their injuries and their lingering effects.

They are battling a deficit of vision about who they are and what they have the ability to do.

Fuck that.

These strong men and women need us to stand beside them as they fight their inner demons. They need us to speak for them where the zombie dope has left them unable to speak for themselves. They need us to support them as they reach for a life after service that is full of health and life and meaning.

So if you love a Warfighter, then open your eyes. See the signs. Fight for life.

And with every resource you have, make sure that the one you love can Live to Tell the story inside. I am counting on you to work with me, fight with me, speak with me. This battle against pharmaceutical induced suicide is too hard for any of us to win alone.

Together we will | MAMA LUTZ

EPILOGUE
NOT AN OPTION

"THE THINGS WE DON'T SAY"

People in our country have been taught that it's bad manners to bring up religion at the dinner table. Politics, religion, and sex – those were the topics you just didn't mention so that no one got upset. Well, I hope you're not eating right now, because we're going to have a talk.

For a great deal of my life, I did not consider Elohim as part of my life. I'll tell you why in a minute. When I was going through the most pain, I accepted as reality the idea that I had to go through it alone. People could be nice to me, but no one else could really share the load that had landed on me.

I have come to understand since then that I was mistaken in that idea. God, he was always with me, and I was just too blind to see. I had too much pride, because I was so independent that I couldn't see him. I'm a doer. I get stuff done. And I'm one of the types of people that has a hard time at times waiting for God to do something when we can get up and we can get it done ourselves. You know what I mean?

Knowing Yahweh for who he is and trusting him to be

there with me in pain has made all the difference. I still feel grief and lose hope sometimes, but I have someone with me in the middle of that trauma. For instance, I have a hard time on the anniversaries, like Johnny's birthday and his last day. Sometimes those dates hit me out of the blue.

Towards the end of last April, I started to feel anxiety in my midsection. I was like, "What is going on? What is this?" Because I know what happens on significant dates, I check for them. Once I realized the cause of my trauma, by the next day it was gone. I could bring it out from hiding and trust it to my Father to handle on my behalf.

For years those dates would affect me sometimes months at a time with varying degrees of depression. Now, if something tries to come on me, I will immediately say no to it. I am not taking that on. I'll either pray or praise and worship. When that blanket of heaviness comes on me, I'll say, "Oh, no, no, no, no – you're not coming on me. Not today, devil!"

I have come to realize through my experience that no matter how much I wanted it to be so, cutting faith out of life was simply not an option.

"WHERE IS THE LOVE?"

Constant church involvement and religious belief should have been the natural path of my life. Even as a child, I was always involved in community. When I was ten years old, I was raising money for Muscular Dystrophy. The Skipper Chuck Show, a local show down here, had a contest on who could raise the most money for MD. I used to knock on people's doors. I would sell avocados on the street corners. I was always doing something. I was the highest money raiser, and I won a trip to Disney World.

I was always saving money so I could buy my mom a Mother's Day present or a Christmas present. I wanted to have the best gifts for my mom. So, I was naturally giving. And just like I am now, I was concerned with other people, serving them and connecting them.

I was raised in the Baptist church, and where I was at that time, it was hell and damnation. I never knew the love of Elohim! What I heard was, "You're a dirty sinner, and you need Jesus. You need to accept him into your heart. All you have to do is believe in him and have him in your heart, and you'll go to heaven."

I did not hear about the incredible love of Yahweh, his acceptance and peace. There was no carrot in that faith, only stick. And there was no encouragement to question what was taught, read the Scriptures, and come up with my own conclusions. Sure, I should read the Bible for myself – as long as I came up with the same ideas as the pastor at the end.

And of course, there was no love in my house. It's like we all got dressed on Sunday, my mom in her pretty dress and my dad in his coat. We would go to church, and we would come home. And then the fighting would start. It lasted all week.

When my dad would come home from work, we'd yell, "Dad's home!" And we'd run to our rooms, because we didn't want to get yelled at. We didn't want to do anything to make him mad.

I turned away from the church for a while. I've been an independent woman all my life. When I put my mind to something, I get it done myself. I didn't see that involvement in church had anything to do with the way I approached life.

But in the nineties, I tried religion again and became very active in church. My children were young, and I wanted to give them a faith. So we went to a small place of worship right by my house. I made a point to know everybody's name, and I said hello to everybody. I hugged everyone! I'm really into community and encouraging people.

Our church would have dinner on a Wednesday night and then have a service. This one Wednesday I said, "I want to cook the whole meal for everybody. I want to do everything from start to finish." That was my heart, to give to them and bless them.

I made a huge tray of baked ziti. I made a salad. I made garlic bread. I made a big pot of rice pudding for dessert. I brought it, and we all ate together. That's just one example of how involved I was in everything.

Then my children's father came down with cancer. And

not one person from that church helped me. Not one person cooked me a meal. Not one came to babysit my kids. Not one.

I needed help; I did not leave my children's father alone in the hospital. I had a home daycare at that time. So, I would spend the night in the hospital while my sister was spending the night at my house. Then in the morning I would go home, and she would go to the hospital and stay with him all day. I would work, and then I would finish my work and go to the hospital. I would just do that around the clock.

And Johnny was so sweet! I'd get back at six in the morning, and I would sleep. Those thoughtful boys tried to let me sleep as much as possible. One morning when I got up, Johnny said, "Mommy, I made Justin breakfast."

I said, "Thank you, honey!" He'd made him peanut butter and jelly so that I could sleep.

He would let me sleep until the first knock on the door. Then he'd wake me up and say, "Mommy, the kids are here."

I'd say, "Okay, honey, thank you." And I'd get up and take care of the daycare kids.

Here my young son, out of the natural goodness of his heart, was doing practical things to show me his care and support. Meanwhile, all these holy people that talked a lot about the love of God just left me out to dry. And so I was done. I was shocked. I just couldn't believe it.

I stayed away from anything traditionally religious for

many years. I could not bring myself to believe that there was anything real to the whole business. The fake people at the church around the corner seemed to be practicing the same faith as my parents. So, I never knew the love of a father until recently.

I beat myself up a lot since I've come to faith for all the years that I was away from Elohim. But I wasn't able to see him at those times for whatever reason. Why now all of the sudden do I have this grand connection to him? Why now, and why not before? Because now is the time he drew me in. Everything is always in his perfect timing.

On the way to work today, I was praise and worshipping, and just a peace and a calm came over me. When you surrender everything to him, you know that nothing is yours. You have nothing. It is all his – both the treasure to share and the pain to handle. It really is so beautiful and so peaceful, and it's such a beautiful thing to be able to trust him.

"There Had to be Something Else"

Last summer, I had thought about suicide again. Faith had not been a part of my journey. I know that my son was very angry at God after he returned from combat, and when I thought about doing the Buddy Up, I looked at everything from my son's point of view. I just wanted to welcome everybody at exactly where they were. I didn't want anybody to think that I was trying to change them. I just wanted to love them exactly where they were.

But I came to the realization this summer, after contemplating suicide, that I was just focusing on the negative. When I really saw the evil that is in the world and how evil man is, then I knew that there is definitely a God. There had to be the opposite of that. There had to be good, and there has to be a God who is the source of that good.

So, I just started listening to praise and worship music, and it really uplifted my spirit. I started to be open to the idea that there was a God. I still was really unsure about things, but I just knew there has to be good from the law of polarity.

I found the music that spoke to me on YouTube, and a recommended video came on from Let Us Worship. I started listening to them. And I just started sobbing before God and praising him and loving him and for the first time just feeling his love. Like I was enveloped by his love, and it was my desire to see Let Us Worship in person.

Randomly I texted an acquaintance: "Hey, you ever heard of Let Us Worship? Sean Feucht?"

She answered, "Yeah, we're going to see him today!"

Incredibly, they were here in West Palm Beach! I was able to go to them for five days in a row! I went to revival. There I met some new friends, and I ended up visiting church again for the first time in years.

I started hearing the Word. And I liked what I was hearing. It was satisfying something in me. At that point, I really started to get into the Word, where I was faithfully reading it every morning. I would get up at five and just start reading it. I was seeing the truth for myself. I didn't need a preacher to tell me what to think.

Now I can't get out of the Word. I get up early in the morning before work. I'm eating it. I feel a hunger that only the Word can satisfy. And I feel that even my expression is different. The expression on my face is softer. I just see that it's changing me from deep within. And only God can do that. Only God can change us so deeply and teach us the truth by his Spirit.

Here is what I know. God is love, and all he wants to do is love us. He wants to transform us. He wants us to love him with all of our heart, our soul, our strength, and our mind. He wants us to love our fellow man. He wants us to take care of the homeless and the widows and the elderly. It's all about love!

And prayer—he wants us to seek him for everything that we do. When we get up in the morning, he wants to be the first thing on our minds. He wants to direct our paths. He wants to protect us. He wants to comfort us.

"Faithfulness"

I've done a lot of change. In my house, I had a lot of Eastern religious symbolism. And I've gotten rid of it all because I look at that stuff as man's copy of God's truth. Like even Christmas, this Friday I got rid of every Christmas decoration that I had in storage. So I don't celebrate any of man's customs anymore.

This is the truth that Yahweh has given me. This is my being true outwardly to what I know inwardly. If this is not your faith path, then embrace the faith that you know inside your heart. That connection to our Father is so important.

I just see that everything good in this world is of God. I give him the glory, and I live for him. That is my only desire, is to serve him and to be a delight in his eyes, to glorify his name, to be a light, to bring others to the kingdom, and just to stand strong in my faith and not to fear. Not to fear, and not to live by sight but live by faith.

Will I still do yoga? Yeah, I'll still do yoga. But when I do it, my mind will be on Yehua. It won't be on myself. Because with my beliefs, and with the parable of the seed, the seed has to die for the fruit that is inside to birth. That's why I try and die to my own flesh daily so that God's fruit can birth and rise up inside me.

Will I still take herbs and teach about them? Of course I will! God gave us all those herbs for healing. So, I grow as many herbs as I can. I also will still fight for our veterans and the rest of America to use Cannabis as the helpful plant it is.

This path of faith is just a journey that I'm on. And I

don't want to force any religion, because I truly believe that God, Father Yehua, he calls us in his perfect time.

I don't believe in using evangelism like some kind of sales talk where I try to convince people that I've got the only ticket out of hell. What I do when I evangelize is sit somewhere where there's a lot of people and wait for somebody to sit next to me. This is with a veteran or with anybody. You just wait, and you make eye contact. You go, "Hey, how are you doing today?" And you just start talking.

Maybe something will come up that you can really start talking about and having a deeper conversation; maybe not. And then when the conversation is ending, I'll usually just say, "Hey, is there anything I can pray about for you?"

We started doing this at the Buddy Up. I have prayer requests now as they register. I give them the card and say, "If you have anything you want me to pray for, just write it down on here."

Prayer is important. God hears our prayers. He hears the cries of our hearts. I think prayer is important specifically for veterans.

You may have someone in your life like my Johnny was, who is not open to faith. Maybe what he or she saw in combat is still a barrier between that person and listening for the call of God. I would say to you, pray for your veteran. He or she needs connection, and so you definitely need to connect them with a local buddy, another veteran who can listen.

Then you need to pray. Pray alone. Continually pray that God would draw your Warfighter into the kingdom, that God would soften your dear one's heart and remove the veil. People can't see God unless he wills because he has a veil over their eyes. It's not time for them to see him sometimes. It wasn't time for me for decades. But as soon as I turned to Yahweh, I found that he had always been there waiting.

Those of us who love a veteran have to stand in the gap for those who don't see. I pray, "Father, they don't understand. Father, I stand in the gap for them. Father, soften their heart, remove the veil from their eyes and their ears, Father, and draw them in."

This is what you can do when nothing else helps. You can turn to Yahweh and pour out your heart. For as long as there have been people, people have acknowledged the power of faith for physical and emotional healing. To refuse this avenue of help is like a climber on a cliff's edge refusing an outstretched hand. It's simply not an option.

ADDENDUM 1
Aftermath

I recently discovered the following essay that Johnny wrote. It was on an old computer. I'm not sure if it was an assignment that Johnny was given or if it was something that he wrote on his own. In either case, it describes Johnny's very private memories of the impact that combat still had on Johnny long after he had come home.

It wasn't until my last hospitalization that I realized that it wasn't just witnessing the loss of my best friend. Until that point, I was very arrogant. I believed that nothing else on the deployment... the watching other friends die, medevacing Marines, the almost daily firefights, etc.... had affected me in a negative way. I think what affected me the most was the constant and unrelenting hate in my heart. Just every day wishing nothing but the worst on the Taliban. Always wanting to hurt them, to make their families feel what I have felt. You have to have it in you all the time, too. Having it in there is why it felt normal to go out every day to shoot at people and be shot at by people.

There are too many fire fights for me to go into all of them, and besides, I saw, smelled, felt, thought, and acted the same way in all of them. It was even the same temp for all of them: hot. So there is really no reason for me to go into detail about all of them except for the parts that I have come to believe have affected me.

I would always be terribly scared that my actions or lack there-of would get Marines killed. I still do believe some things were my fault. Every step of every patrol, I feared that someone was going to be killed and that I would have to watch someone else bleed out, watch their eyes turn lifeless. That is a horrible feeling, always wondering who is going to be next.

One of the most traumatic experiences for me happened on 07-23-09.

Whenever we were leaving on a foot patrol, a friend of mine named Davila and I had a ritual. We would catch each other, and he would say to me, "Don't get shot." In return, if he was going out on a mobile patrol (because he was on the mobile section), I would say, "Don't get blown up."

My squad happened to go out on a patrol, and Davila and I exchanged our usual goodbyes. We were out for hours on the foot patrol because we had received a little bit of contact. On our way back, we could see the mobile section leave the COP going down a parallel road. No sooner had the Humvees gotten out of sight than my friend was saying they needed to slow down. Then we heard an IED going off. Since we were already out, we got there first to secure the area.

Once we got there, I didn't think that anyone had survived. Then I heard Davila screaming because his leg and foot were gone. The Humvee looked as if it was a sardine can. The engine block was 150mm away, along with the turret and glass. It took us a while to get there; so the medics had already taken care of the KIAs.

Once the Blackhawks landed, a friend and I picked up a body bag. When we did, we jerked it because it was so light; we were expecting to be heavier. We looked inside it. It was Jeremy Lasher. Lasher and I had gone to SOI together, and I had been with him since coming to 2/8. It wasn't really even Lasher, just his torso. Once the birds left, we had to get in line and pick up what was left of Lasher.

One of the other traumatic times in my life was when my squad occupied OP Empire. It was not like the other OPs. When Empire got attacked, it really got attacked. It was common knowledge that the Taliban wanted to overrun that OP. We never found out why they wanted the OP gone so much. Every day we would hear them talk about getting in new computer guidance software so that they could aim the 107mm rockets that they already always launched at us better.

It's a hard thing to look at your buds and tell them that we won't get captured, that we will kill each other first. There were only 13 of us there to defend against up to 75 Taliban fighters from a distance of 1000 to 40mm away. With no reinforcements, the only things we had were air and fire support. Standing post at night, all you could hear was the Marines screaming in their sleep because of the night terror of being overrun. At the end of our time there, we had all changed. Nobody can experience that much fear and be the same.

On 09-26-09, we were going on a long-range patrol. The objective was not to take contact but to try to get eyes on the town of Lakari and the market there that we had plans on taking over. The only support the squad took was us, the machine gunners. Right before we had gotten there, the Taliban opened up on us.

I was in the rear of the patrol. The patrol had been up against the embankment of a canal. We then jumped the canal to get up on the road to return fire. That's when we heard Marines yelling for a Corpsman. Jared and I jumped back down to get closer to the squad. In the midst of this, we had separated ourselves a little. Once we got closer, we saw that the casualty was Jordan Chrobot.

We had set up a 360, and then out of nowhere the fire stopped. Two "civilians" walked right up to where we were to get a better idea of our location and then turned around and walked back. Then, of course, the fire returned, except a lot more accurate. Then the bird came in, but didn't land and flew away, because another squad 2 km away just got hit by an IED.

So our bird came in taking fire, and they put Chrobot on the bird. But you could just see death, it was painfully easy to spot. We knew that he was going nowhere. At this point, the company had to send another squad to back us up. I had already run out of 7.62 for my 240.

I really don't know what else to talk about. I don't want to bring up more fire fights. They were all the same. Dead Marines are dead Marines. So is getting shot at, shooting at people, and seeing dead children. It's all the same. It's terrible.

ADDENDUM 2
The Plan

I found this document on the old computer as well. I'm not sure why or when Johnny wrote it. What is obvious to me, however, is that Johnny had a very detailed plan. And that plan was to live.

Once going home awaiting orders, I will work at the family business. The business is called "Super Stone". We manufacture everything for decorative concrete: sealers, acid stains, color hardeners, release agents, concrete stamps, and much more.

I will work there until my schooling starts on January 5th at Palm Beach State College. I have already applied to the school. Once accepted, I will enroll myself into their Commercial Pilot College Credit Course. There are no prerequisites for this course. However, I will have to take a placement test and score well to enroll in the course. The course will take three semesters. I will receive my Private Pilot's License, Instrument Rating, and Commercial License.

The second half of my schooling will begin in the spring of 2013. The course is the Professional Pilot Track for the Associate of Science Degree. This is an eighteen-month course. When I am finished with the course, I will have an Associate of Science Professional Pilot degree. I will also have these other licenses: Flight

Instructor, Flight Instructor Instrument, Commercial Pilot NVG Flight, Commercial Pilot External Load, and Commercial Pilot Turbine Flight.

Once completing school, I will work at the family business again while I try to get a job as a helicopter pilot.

PHOTO
GALLERY

(The following are a few photos of Johnny in Afghanisgtan and when he came back)

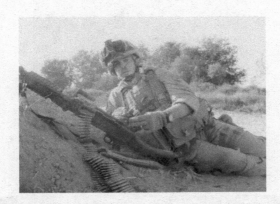

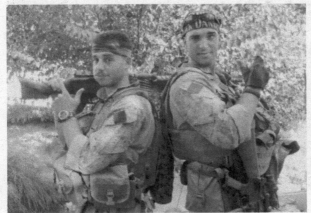

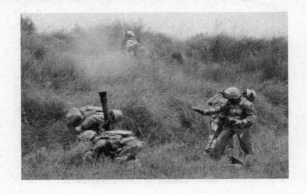

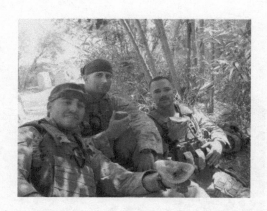

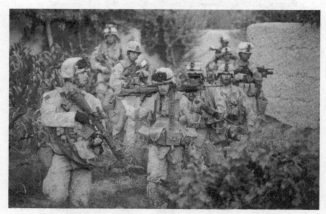

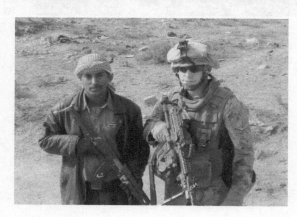

236

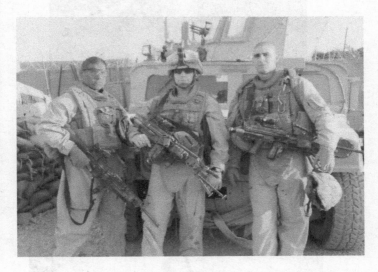

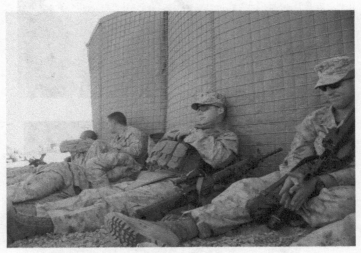

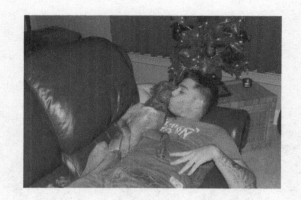

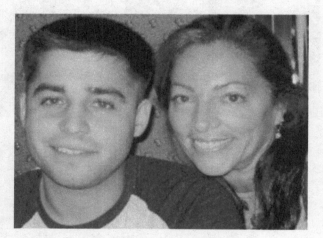

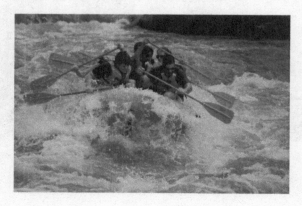

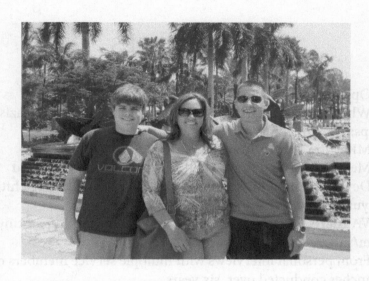

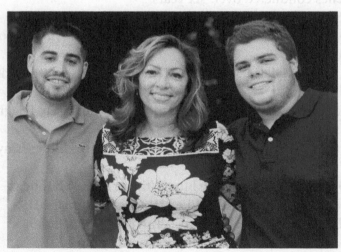

239

ENDNOTES

1, Operation Paperclip | https://tinyurl.com/gq9hua9

2, What Cold War CIA Interrogators Learned from the Nazis | https://tinyurl.com/yd7qj58a

3, MK-Ultra | https://tinyurl.com/yd7qj58a

4, Mefloquine (Oral Route) | https://tinyurl.com/y9kdhzud

5, Development of Mefloquine As an Antimalarial Drug | https://tinyurl.com/y9hsabkp

6, VA Alerts Doctors to Malaria-Drug Concerns | https://tinyurl.com/yawresoh

7, From personal interviews with multiple service members of all branches conducted over six years

8, A Serious Nightmare | https://tinyurl.com/yctchg7r

9, Psychiatric Side Effects of Mefloquine | https://tinyurl.com/yctchg7r'

10, ... Anti-Malarial... Isn't in Medical Records | https://tinyurl.com/yytmhzwd

11, Your First Step in Recovery Is to Get an Accurate Diagnosis | https://tinyurl.com/yakexz8z

12, Interview with Commander Bill Manofsky | https://tinyurl.com/yd3coj98

13, Dr. Remington Nevin | https://tinyurl.com/ybnhbgax

14, Phone interview with Mike Lichtenstein, April 2019.

15, Hoffmann-La Roche | https://tinyurl.com/ya9nth5r

16, Leo Sternbach | https://tinyurl.com/cojuflu

17, Chlordiazepoxide | https://tinyurl.com/bwjrmeq

18, Benzodiazepine | https://tinyurl.com/cd3ffr2

19, The Brain from Top to Bottom: Synapses | https://tinyurl.com/yydonnd4

20, Before You Fill That Benzo Description: READ THIS... | https://tinyurl.com/ya9u5gjv

21, Self-Harm and Suicide Associated with Benzodiazepine Use | https://tinyurl.com/ybm7aq66

22, Xanax, Valium Tied to Higher Suicide Risk for Some | https://tinyurl.com/ybaxbrp4

23, Prescription Opioid, Benzodiazepine Misuse... | https://tinyurl.com/yan2s7b7

24, Benzodiazepine Users with PTSD... | https://tinyurl.com/yc7srer5

25, Clonazepam | https://tinyurl.com/ycy2u2ho

26, Understanding What Occurs in a Benzodiazepine Overdose | https://tinyurl.com/y8s82t85

27, Klonopin | https://tinyurl.com/y9muxbhv

28, Association with Opioid and Benzodiazepine Misuse... | https://tinyurl.com/yb5553wr

29, Stories of Suicide: Shed Light on Benzodiazepine | https://tinyurl.com/y94oq6vk

30, Suicide: Benzodiazepine Withdrawal Syndrome (BWS) | https://tinyurl.com/yddorbdj

31, A Prescription for Addiction | https://tinyurl.com/ydg8yu7

32, Virginia Doctor Who Prescribed More Than 500,000 Doses... | https://tinyurl.com/yyrpqth8

33, Johnson & Johnson Settles with Two Ohio Counties | https://tinyurl.com/yy3v6nqb

34, Purdue Pharma to Stay in Business... | https://tinyurl.com/y4svbns8

35, Prescription Opioids DrugFacts| https://tinyurl.com/y8e4z687

36, Opioid | https://tinyurl.com/ca56tyo

37, Opioid (Narcotic) Pain Medications | https://tinyurl.com/yc-glmssp

38, Opioid | https://tinyurl.com/ca56tyo

39, Depression and Opioid Use Go Hand in Hand | https://tinyurl.com/ycsbl4sg

40, Drug Deaths in America Are Rising Faster Than Ever | https://tinyurl.com/ybecsysy

41, Understanding the Epidemic | https://tinyurl.com/h9qlzj9

42, Deadly Fentanyl Bought Online from China | https://tinyurl.com/yxfsl2u5

43, Origins of an Epidemic Purdue Pharma Knew... | https://tinyurl.com/yy58y28x

44, The Family That Built an Empire of Pain | https://tinyurl.com/yctwzbbu

45, Purdue Pharma to Stay in Business | https://tinyurl.com/y4svbns8

46, Children of the Opioid Epidemic Are Flooding Foster Homes... | https://tinyurl.com/y8lhxrgv

47, Coroner Reports 10 Overdose Deaths in 26-Hour Period | https://tinyurl.com/y5rdwf45

48, Another Shocking Opioid Statistic | https://tinyurl.com/ybsu4br9

49, A Doctor's Thoughts on the Opioid Epidemic: Anna Lembke | https://tinyurl.com/y5flytef

50, Klonopin | https://tinyurl.com/yytgp22p

51, Phone interview with Kevin Ullman April 2019.

52, Older Vets Committing Suicide at Alarming Rate | https://tinyurl.com/y3sec2av

53, The Real Numbers of Warriors We Are Losing to PTS... | https://tinyurl.com/yyj6f3ow

54, Ketwig: More Veterans Commit Suicide... | https://tinyurl.com/y63gjfub

55, Deaths from Drugs and Suicide Reach a Record in the U.S. | https://tinyurl.com/y64dyowy

56, I Survived Combat in Iraq and a Suicide Attempt at Home | https://tinyurl.com/y6g9jk9a

57, Mom of Veteran Who Died by Suicide | https://tinyurl.com/y2rvs2y9

58, Phone interview with Nicholas Rizzo April 2019.

59, A Young Afghan Pianist Plays for His Country's Future | https://tinyurl.com/y6b8d8mw

60, Rising Young Afghan Pianist Wants World to See | https://tinyurl.com/y37m9kof

61, Personal letter forwarded to me April 9, 2019 from Elham Fanous.

62, Spartan Pledge | https://tinyurl.com/yy88pdlo

63, The Spartan Pledge | https://tinyurl.com/y2ynxmg4

64, Taking the Spartan Pledge Against Suicide | https://tinyurl.com/yyx3hlqx

65, Veterans Vow to Fight Suicide with a Sword | https://tinyurl.com/y5xtxeqq

66, The 9/11 Spartan Sword; Forged to End Veteran Suicide | https://tinyurl.com/yyerv9wz

67, Spartan Pledge: The Oath That Can Defeat Suicide | https://tinyurl.com/y4ckboja

68, The Uniformed Firefighters Association of New York | https://tinyurl.com/y3wn2toj

69, Spartan Pledge Day | https://tinyurl.com/y6e8fqs3

70, Spartan Pledge Day | https://tinyurl.com/y4drf93t

71, Spartan Pledge Event | https://tinyurl.com/y44hlesc

72, Spartan Pledge Day at the VA: Focusing on Veteran Suicide | https://tinyurl.com/y4hxyxpl

73, Phone Interview with Danielle Glaviano April 2019.

74, Phone interview with Mike Lichtenstein April 2019.

75, Health Insurance Portability and Accountability Act | https://tinyurl.com/9tmdtzd

76, What Is a HIPAA Violation? | https://tinyurl.com/ybu9z75g

77, What Is HIPAA and What Does It Regulate? | https://tinyurl.com/yx8hfmbv

78, HIPAA | https://tinyurl.com/y93szexb

79, Your Rights Under HIPAA | https://tinyurl.com/jxezquc

80, How the Discovery of CTE Shifted Thinking | https://tinyurl.com/yy5bvmka

81, Traumatic Brain Injury | https://tinyurl.com/uf2l8dl

82, Traumatic Brain Injury | https://tinyurl.com/y42kzogg

83, Causes and Effects of Traumatic Brain Injury | https://tinyurl.com/y4ubn4ws

84, What Are the Potential Effects of TBI | https://tinyurl.com/y7qsz9rg

85, Traumatic Brain Injury | https://tinyurl.com/yddruqdd

86, Mild Traumatic Brain Injury in U.S. Soldiers | https://tinyurl.com/y6xx7bqz

87, The Epidemiology and Impact of Traumatic Brain Injury | https://tinyurl.com/y4uvujsm

88, Community Integration for Persons | https://tinyurl.com/y3k-sngse

89, Suicide Warning Signs | https://tinyurl.com/yydoddw4

90, What Are Suicidal Thoughts | https://tinyurl.com/y6brevoj

91, Suicidal Behavior | https://tinyurl.com/y9zo67ad

92, Signs & Symptoms of Suicidal Ideation | https://tinyurl.com/yyn2r87x

93, Suicide Risk Factors | https://tinyurl.com/y4rcykn2

94, Recognizing Suicidal Behavior | https://tinyurl.com/y6p6pye4

95, Warning Signs of Suicide | https://tinyurl.com/y3z4lnvy

96, Veterans | https://tinyurl.com/y7jkdjkh

97, Personal interview, May 2019.

98, Your VA Transition Assistance Program (TAP) | https://tinyurl.com/yd6lgkkx

99, Transition Assistance Program (TAP) | https://tinyurl.com/y5l3mu9f

100, Air Force Cuts Back Transition Training Requirements | https://tinyurl.com/y6krndkn

101, Transition Assistance Program (TAP) | https://tinyurl.com/y5cn8kze

102, Transition Readiness | https://tinyurl.com/y3wlbbbb

103, Military Transition Assistance Program | https://tinyurl.com/y2q3d8dg

104, Transition Assistance Programs and Resources | https://tinyurl.com/y287w3zu

105, What Happens During the Transition Assistance Program | https://tinyurl.com/y5w7djwo

106, Military Job Assistance Programs | https://tinyurl.com/y5tafphv

107, Transition Assistance Program | https://tinyurl.com/y63cmh26

108, TAP Is Getting a Makeover This Year | https://tinyurl.com/y4urb45j

109, Changes Coming | https://tinyurl.com/yxhu6w96

110, VA, Army, Navy, and Marines | https://tinyurl.com/y34rqcgc

111, What Is Charlie Mike? | https://tinyurl.com/y67t5hs8

112, Charlie Mike: An Attitude of Action | https://tinyurl.com/yys96v2n

113, The Mission Continues | https://tinyurl.com/yxqld52y

114, Continue Mission: No Veteran Left Behind | https://tinyurl.com/y32dyvnr

115, Continue Mission: Transitioning from the Battlefield | https://tinyurl.com/yy3c4hm9

116, Be Ready to Raise Your Right Hand | https://tinyurl.com/

y57qscj3

117, Letter to Soldiers Being Discharged Following World War II | https://tinyurl.com/yy8la25l

118, Why Veterans Should Continue | https://tinyurl.com/y4owo3a3

119, I Found a Home in Military Green | https://tinyurl.com/y249v4xz

120, Helping People, Changing Lives | https://tinyurl.com/rj8m-r8f

121, Volunteering May Be Good for Body and Mind | https://tinyurl.com/y8u9zeck

122, Volunteering and Its Surprising Benefits | https://tinyurl.com/y3vrygca

123, Volunteering and Health Benefits in General Adults | https://tinyurl.com/y5uhbpsg

124, Connected Warriors Founders | https://tinyurl.com/y23yp-gun

125, From Connected Warriors, personal email September 15, 2019.

126, Transformational Breath | https://tinyurl.com/y2raruv5

127, Dr. Judith Kravitz, personal email September 18, 2019.

128, Exercise: Seven Benefits of Regular Physical Activity | https://tinyurl.com/ybn4tflx

129, 10 Amazing Benefits of Exercise | https://tinyurl.com/y5o77wyo

130, 11 Benefits of Exercise | https://tinyurl.com/yxkr4539

131, Unexpected Benefits of Exercise | https://tinyurl.com/y4rsk-9by

132, What Is Warrior Culture? | https://tinyurl.com/y3l64dg5

133, Developing a Warrior Mindset | https://tinyurl.com/yyqy-drxx

134, Warrior Mindset: Train Your Brain | https://tinyurl.com/

yys7n4do

135, 10 of the Greatest Ancient Warrior Cultures | https://tinyurl.com/y4rbjjtn

136, Living Well with a Disability | https://tinyurl.com/t6vwmhl

137, Disability and Health Information for People with Disabilities | https://tinyurl.com/ydwsq8t5

138, How to Enhance Daily Life for a Person with a Disability | https://tinyurl.com/y6xjgnqa

139, How to Move Forward in Life When You Feel Stuck | https://tinyurl.com/y5lut744

140, How to Break Through Your Inner Limitations | https://tinyurl.com/y53u8th8

141, What I Know About Living With Both | https://tinyurl.com/yxb9jn6w

142, Living with Depression and Addiction | https://tinyurl.com/y4sp8ec9

143, Living with a Mental Health Condition | https://tinyurl.com/yc5xgp33

144, How Drugs Affect Your Body | https://tinyurl.com/y4bsn4ka

145, Effects of Illegal Drugs on the Heart | https://tinyurl.com/y2dafkmz

146, Partnership to End Addiction | https://tinyurl.com/yxknovp9

147, Effects of Drug Addiction | https://tinyurl.com/yxdzfrzt

148, The Effects of Alcohol on Your Body | https://tinyurl.com/y73wcgtk

149, Alcohol's Effect on the Body | https://tinyurl.com/ycjtsfxm

150, Health Risks of Chronic Heavy Drinking | https://tinyurl.com/y52ptgl3

151, Sorting Out the Health Effects of Alcohol | https://tinyurl.com/y7tf98o4

152, Short-Term, Long-Term Effects of Alcohol | https://tinyurl.

com/y5bvhpay

153, Alcohol Use and Your Health | https://tinyurl.com/y2889a7d

154, The Truth ABout 7 Common Food Additives | https://tinyurl.com/yb9f3sbe

155, Food Additives and Human Health | https://tinyurl.com/yaamxkxh

156, Top 10 Food Additives to Avoid | https://tinyurl.com/yxnhb-kxt

157, Top 15 Chemical Additives in Your Food | https://tinyurl.com/slxp9xb

158, 12 Common Food Additives |https://tinyurl.com/y4u-+b-3mal

159, Common Food Additives and Chemicals| https://tinyurl.com/y64ch6pu

160, Analysis Confirms Chemicals in Food Are More Hazardous | https://tinyurl.com/y3r3mhn5

161, 6 Reasons to Drink Water | https://tinyurl.com/ya2egml6

162, 7 Science-Based Health Benefits of Drinking Enough Water | https://tinyurl.com/y8k7e9cy

163, 10 Unexpected Reasons to Drink More Water | https://tinyurl.com/yb87qk9e

164, 10 Reasons Why You Should Drink More Water | https://tinyurl.com/y8vcznw3

165, Fifteen Benefits of Drinking Water | https://tinyurl.com/yauaslgd

166, The Benefits of Eating Fresh | https://tinyurl.com/y2jwtb7w

167, Why Is Eating Healthy | https://tinyurl.com/y67bnqk7

168, Vegetables | https://tinyurl.com/y532s6em

169, Healthy Eating | https://tinyurl.com/y9nv78sd

170, Let Food Be Thy Medicine | https://tinyurl.com/y2ytfuz5

171, 5 Foods You Should Be Eating for Your Best Body | https://tinyurl.com/y2rkozgp

172, 50 Foods That Are Super Healthy | https://tinyurl.com/y8jc-jmyq

173, Eating Healthy | https://tinyurl.com/yxe6q5b6

174, 6 Natural Sleep Remedies |https://tinyurl.com/ycysvfoc

175, 14 Natural Remedies to Beat Insomnia | https://tinyurl.com/y2yxvume

176, 5 Natural Herbs Guaranteed to Help You Sleep | https://tinyurl.com/y2czggy3

177, The 6 Best Herbs That Help You Sleep | https://tinyurl.com/y2b9wko2

178, 6 Natural Herbs That Help You Fall Asleep Instantly | https://tinyurl.com/y3r3g52c

179, 8 Natural Remedies That Will May Help You Sleep | https://tinyurl.com/y4gemfxt

180, 6 Herbs and Supplements for Depression | https://tinyurl.com/y9y7sx3n

181, 8 Natural Depression Remedies to Consider | https://tinyurl.com/yxzreyeq

182, Natural Remedies for Depression | https://tinyurl.com/y6o97cjn

183, 11 Natural Treatments for Depression | https://tinyurl.com/yyac87wb

184, 15 Incredible Natural Remedies for Anxiety and Depression | https://tinyurl.com/yyfhnh4n

185, 10 Natural Depression Treatments | https://tinyurl.com/y5qmr2v8

186, 7 Natural Remedies for Stress and Anxiety | https://tinyurl.com/yyc2srcz

187, Anxiety and Stress Relief| https://tinyurl.com/y5gegz6p

188, Anxiety Natural Remedies | https://tinyurl.com/qm5rcu4

189, Proven Natural Remedies for Anxiety | https://tinyurl.com/y56p6j8v

190, 10 Trusted Home Remedies for Natural Anxiety Relief | https://tinyurl.com/y29w7kak

191, How to Treat Anxiety Naturally | https://tinyurl.com/y6l-s33kj

192, 5 Surprising Natural Painkillers | https://tinyurl.com/yy-gorfqn

193, 6 Natural Remedies for Conquering Chronic Pain | https://tinyurl.com/y4etthkj

194, 14 Drug-Free Ways to Ease Chronic Pain | https://tinyurl.com/y2rt3xgn

195, Natural Remedies for Chronic Pain | https://tinyurl.com/yyrmj8z5

196, 6 Cheap, Natural, and Quick Chronic Pain Remedies | https://tinyurl.com/y79xfcvd

197, Natural Home Remedy Treatments | https://tinyurl.com/y3charq5

198, Alternative Treatments for Chronic Pain | https://tinyurl.com/yx9bn5os

199, The Racist Origins of Marijuana Prohibition | https://tinyurl.com/ydfkqdtd

200, 33 Examples | https://tinyurl.com/yxls5q4g

201, The Mysterious History of "Marijuana" | https://tinyurl.com/yc4deq6s

202, Medical Marijuana | https://tinyurl.com/yyd9ymbx

203, Medical Marijuana Treatment |https://tinyurl.com/y9f6ba3p

204, Colorado Family Physicians' Attitudes | https://tinyurl.com/y585vfbp

205, Medical Marijuana FAQ | https://tinyurl.com/y9h3qwft

206, Does CBD Oil Work for Chronic Pain Management? | https://tinyurl.com/yxmyu933

207, Cannabidiol (CBD): What We Know and What We Don't | https://tinyurl.com/y43y3gzk

208, 7 Benefits and Uses of CBD Oil | https://tinyurl.com/y445w-j3e

209, CBD Oil | https://tinyurl.com/ybsdv5nk

210, Personal conversation with Boone Cutler, March 30, 2019.

RESOURCES

Complex PTSD: From Surviving to Thriving
by Pete Walker

Waking the Tiger: Healing Trauma
by Peter A. Levine

*Trauma and Recovery: The Aftermath of Violence -
From Domestic Abuse to Political Terror*
by Judith Lewis Herman

*It Didn't Start with You: How Inherited Family Trauma Shapes
Who We Are and How to End the Cycle*
by Mark Wolynn

Breath: The New Science of a Lost Art
by James Nestor

When the Body Says No: The Cost of Hidden Stress
by Gabor Maté

*In an Unspoken Voice: How the Body Releases Trauma
and Restores Goodness*
by Peter A. Levine

Wintering: The Power of Rest and Retreat in Difficult Times
by Katherine May

251

Maybe You Should Talk to Someone: A Therapist, Her Therapist, and Our Lives Revealed
by Lori Gottlieb

How to Do the Work: Recognize Your Patterns, Heal from Your Past, and Create Your Self
by Nicole LePera

Group: How One Therapist and a Circle of Strangers Saved My Life
by Christie Tate

Burnout: The Secret to Unlocking the Stress Cycle
by Emily Nagoski

The Deepest Well: Healing the Long-Term Effects of Childhood Adversity
by Nadine Burke Harris

The Body Is Not an Apology: The Power of Radical Self-Love
by Sonya Renee Taylor

The Body Keeps the Score: Brain, Mind, and Body in the Healing of Trauma
by Bessel van der Kolk

The Holy Bible

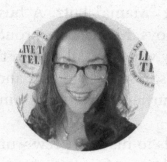

About the Author

Americans have gotten good at military homecomings. After the national shame and scarring that Vietnam Vets endured, the American public changed its heart and welcomed home veterans of the Gulf War, Iraq, and Afghanistan. But in recent years, it has become increasingly apparent that parades and barbeques aren't enough.

Americans have lost more veterans to suicide in the past twenty years than all the Americans we lost in World War I. That's three times the number we lost in Vietnam and six times the number of patriots who died in the American Revolution.

The military is a small proportion of the American population, so chances are that most people don't know a servicemember personally. More of them might know a veteran (from a distance). Those who mourn the losses of service members and veterans to suicide are relatively small in number. But they don't have the luxury of turning away. So they're doing something.

One of those people taking on the tragedy of veteran suicide is Janine "Mama" Lutz. A businesswoman and mother of two boys, Mama Lutz proudly supported her older son Johnny when he enlisted in the Marines. After two deployments, one to Iraq and another to Afghanistan, Johnny returned home with minor injuries to his body.

But the wounds to his soul grew worse and worse under the VA regimen of opioids and benzodiazepines. Far from soothing his sadness and anxiety, the VA-prescribed pharmaceuticals left Johnny unable to process his feelings or retain joy. Most heinously, it pushed thoughts of suicide into his mind until he could no longer resist them.

Johnny Lutz, a cheerful, brave, energetic man, died from Pharmaceutical Induced Suicide (PIS) in 2013. Wracked by grief and haunted by the memory of finding his brother's body, Johnny's brother Justin also died of suicide in 2015. Their deaths devastated their mother.

But she did not shut herself away in grief. A year after Johnny's death, she established an annual memorial ride from his high school to a local park to raise awareness of veteran suicide. Shortly afterward, she established *The LCpl Janos V. Lutz Live to Tell Foundation* in her son's honor.

Live to Tell has provided Janine with practical ways to combat the suicide epidemic. Through *Lutz Buddy Up Social Clubs*, Mama Lutz provides a welcoming space for veterans and first-responders to connect with each other, form friendships and talk about the things they have experienced that civilians can't understand. Another function of *Live to Tell* is the #IwasLutz page, where Mama Lutz collects the stories of many veterans who battled the VA-prescribed pharmaceuticals—some successfully and others not. *Live to Tell* also sponsors the *Vet Connect Mobile App*, utilized by first responders to connect veterans to each other quickly and efficiently to prevent suicides.

In addition to all of her work with the foundation and her full-time job, Mama Lutz also advocates for cannabis decriminalization, legalization, and deschedulization. After thorough research and first-hand experience with a multitude of veterans, she knows the benefits of cannabis for veterans with PTS. In fact, she insists that her son, Johnny, would be living today had he been given the option of cannabis instead of VA-prescribed pharmaceuticals.

In order to spread the word about veteran suicide and the options she has found to stop it, Mama Lutz regularly speaks around her home state of Florida and other places in the US. She has also written *Live to Tell* to tell her son's story and help other military families deal with PTS in a healthy and effective way.

pharmaceutical-induced suicide \ n

1: death by suicide directly caused by neurotoxic chemicals within prescription drugs that derail personal choice and healthy thought | 2: death caused by prescription drugs hijacking a person's will and thought process | 3: the self-inflicted death of a patient induced by the medication they are prescribed | 4: the cause of such a death by negligence of the prescriber

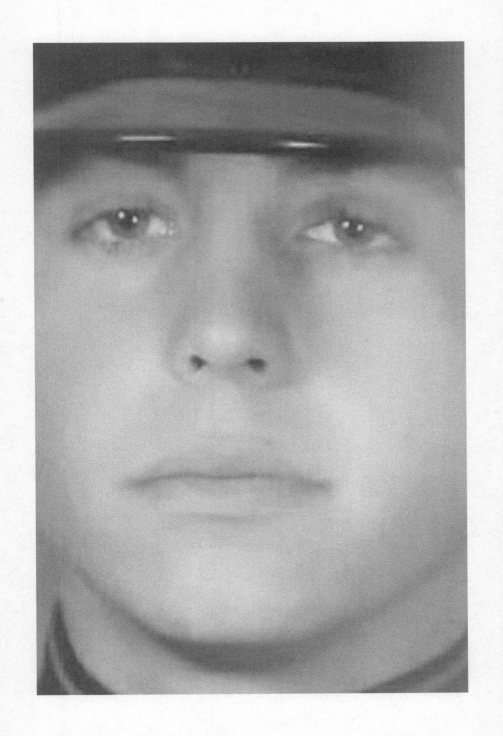

CPSIA information can be obtained
at www.ICGtesting.com
Printed in the USA
LVHW030340170921
698019LV00005B/21